More Praise for
THE BREAST CANCER ANSWERS BOOK

"*The Breast Cancer Answers Book* takes the uncertainty and guesswork out of understanding complex medical terms. You can hear the warmth, care and insight in Jay's and Phyllis's writing, which leaves readers feeling encouraged to work through these difficult times. Definitely an excellent read!"

—Lisa A. Ekman, breast cancer survivor, Ekman Associates

"*The Breast Cancer Answers Book* provides a unique perspective for both the survivor and the provider. The tools to prepare for the breast cancer journey, its discussion of decision making, treatment options, physical and emotional recovery, and survivorship issues provide a practical and thoughtful resource for survivors and their caregivers."

—Jennifer R. Klemp, PhD, MPH, Founder/CEO, Cancer Survivorship Training, University of Kansas Medical Center

D1417350

More About
THE BREAST CANCER ANSWERS BOOK

Based upon decades of patient treatment and medical expertise—for the first time in a how-to source co-authored by patient and physician—*The Breast Cancer Answers Book* **offers you wisdom** into how "breast cancer" is in fact a variety of diseases, insight into your specific form of breast cancer, why time is your friend, your treatment choices, the roles of each doctor and professional on your medical team, and the **power you possess** in treating your disease and your body.

Answer your unasked question.

Just as you may be treated so that your breast is surgically reconstructed—how may you achieve Emotional Reconstruction® over breast cancer? Here for the first time is your answer.

THE
BREAST
CANCER
ANSWERS
BOOK

Author Bios

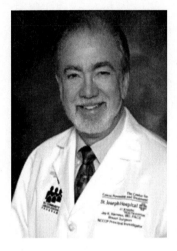 **JAY K. HARNESS, MD, FACS,** a past president of The American Society of Breast Surgeons and Breast Surgery International, works full time in private practice as a breast surgeon in Orange, California. He currently serves as a clinical professor of surgery at University of California, Irvine. For twenty-eight years, Dr. Harness worked in full-time academic general surgery at institutions such as the University of Michigan, Tufts University, the University of California, Davis, and the University of California, San Francisco.

For the past three decades, Dr. Harness has advocated for a multidisciplinary team approach to the treatment of breast cancer. He served as the founding medical director of the University of Michigan's Breast Care Center (BCC) in 1985. The Michigan BCC became one the first academic multidisciplinary breast cancer programs in the United States. His first book, *Breast Cancer: Collaborative Management,* promoted multidisciplinary care. Subsequently, Dr. Harness established and directed similar breast cancer programs in Boston and Orange, California.

In 2011 Dr. Harness cofounded Breast Cancer Answers (breastcanceranswers.com), a website designed for patients and their families. This site introduced the first social media program for breast cancer patients, and it provides information from breast cancer experts that can be accessed anonymously and for free. Visitors will find a searchable library of informative videos with answers to questions raised by women with breast cancer.

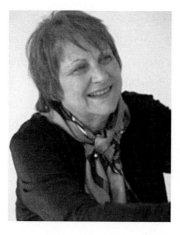

PHYLLIS GAPEN was a Houston-based journalist who survived breast cancer for twenty-four years. She worked to help generate a vision of how new technology, clinical research, creatively organized medical care, and human compassion can push forward science and medical practice.

For more than fifteen years, Phyllis worked with a university team whose engineers helped build advanced Internets for educational and research efforts in Texas. Among other things, that work improved the commodity Internet used by the public. These efforts enabled better transmission of sound and pictures over the Internet, eliminating jerky movements in video playback, and paving the way for popular sites such as YouTube. Better networks also assisted health care professionals in bringing innovations to the practice of medicine. The video-based

Continued Author Bios

breast cancer website Breast Cancer Answers is just one example of such advances.

During her career, Phyllis published more than 100 articles in national publications, including *The Wall Street Journal.* She edited three books, and her work has been cited in fifteen books on health and science policy.

Phyllis often wrote about groups of patients who have difficulty advocating for themselves. She dreamed of a time when cancer therapies would be less toxic, and large numbers of patients would go on to live long, productive lives.

THE BREAST CANCER ANSWERS BOOK

Your Guide to Achieving
Emotional Reconstruction®

JAY K. HARNESS, M.D.
and PHYLLIS GAPEN, B.A.

This book is dedicated to

the women and men

whose lives are changed forever

by the diagnosis of breast cancer.

You are not alone.

We are all in this together.

Together we will triumph.

We Live You®

Contents

Many Thanks

We wish to thank our colleagues, our patients, and others who lovingly reviewed the contents of this book and gave us their invaluable input:

Blynn Bunney, PhD
Michele Carpenter, MD
Norma Castro
Stacy Ferrante, RN
Afshin Forouzannia, MD
Wendy Hartley
Rita Jones
Shu-Yuan Liao, MD
Maria Lopez-Carale, RPT
David Margileth, MD
Mynde Mayfield
Alice Rodriguez, RN

Introduction

Breast cancer greatly impacts the lives of women, changing their lives forever. From the moment a woman receives a breast cancer diagnosis, she begins a physically and emotionally challenging journey.

In the beginning, no map exists for her unique and personal journey. A woman takes the first steps on her own, cautiously testing her footing on a road on which she feels vulnerable. As she adapts to her new reality, she taps her inner resources and turns to special guides who will accompany her on her healing journey.

Some of these guides are people she'll come to know well. Others she'll never meet. They are all part of the large medical team that will map out a personalized plan for treating her cancer and then accompany her on what will become a lifelong journey. This plan will be individualized to her medical situation.

Her experience will illustrate the dawning of an era, and medical revelations that promise to change the paradigm of breast cancer treatment. A one-size-fits-all approach will no longer be the norm. This book provides a guide to the new breast cancer treatments made possible through scientific achievements. In simple language, it explains the steps that breast cancer patients will take along a path that leads to the execution of a personalized treatment plan. That plan evolves from the use of a multidisciplinary approach to the diagnosis and treatment of breast cancer.

Such plans include steps for treatment and follow-up, screening for recurrence, dealing with treatment side effects, and adapting to a lifelong status as a cancer survivor.

This book was written in partnership with the team from Breast Cancer Answers (breastcanceranswers.com), including an experienced breast cancer surgeon and a twenty-four-year breast cancer survivor. The book is packed with information— and regularly augmented with emerging data about breast cancer developments published on the website, which keeps patients and their families informed.

In the future, women's breast cancer experiences will change, reflecting progress in diagnosis and treatment. This book maps the paths now possible for the healing journeys women will undertake which results in achieving *Emotional Reconstruction.*®

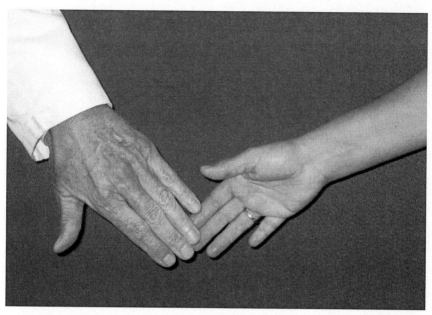

Reaching for your hand, let us begin the journey together.
You are not alone.

Chapter 1

Time Is Our Friend: Taking Time to Plan Treatment Before Surgery

Women who discover that cancer is growing in their breasts want to get rid of it. Many of them want to do so quickly—today, tomorrow, no later than next week.

But rushing into surgery without taking the time to gather sufficient information about the particular cancer often complicates matters. Hurrying can lead to extra operations and undesirable outcomes that neither the surgeon nor the patient want.

Planning surgery takes time. Many steps lead up to the physician and the patient making good, shared decisions about modern, individualized care that combats tumors. Carefully considered choices can lead to better outcomes and better quality of life after treatment. In some cases, planning helps reduce the severity of the measures required to treat the cancer.

Several decades ago, patients newly diagnosed with breast cancer were quickly taken into an operating room for surgery. But today's tools enable physicians to tailor treatments for individual patients. Devising such personalized treatment requires that doctors gather information about an individual, and about her specific breast cancer.

Today's surgeons look at mammograms, breast MRIs (magnetic resonance imaging), ultrasound studies, and the pathology results of core needle biopsies. They also consider the woman's breast size and her preferred choices among treatments. Before a surgeon steps inside the operating suite, he or she talks to the patient about breast conservation versus mastectomy.

Following the planning steps used by a surgeon provides insight into this intense process.

"In my practice in Orange, I like to tell my patients that time is our friend," explains California breast surgeon Jay Harness, MD. "What do I mean by that? I am conveying a high intention: the patient and I want to go to the operating room only once, and we want to know exactly what we're going to do in the operating room. We want to know that what we're planning to do in the OR meets the patient's needs and provides good cancer treatment.

"While my patients are waiting to set a date for surgery, I ask them to embrace their cancer mentally, emotionally, and spiritually. This involves accepting the reality that a tumor exists, and marshaling internal resources to face that reality and undergo treatment. Doing so will prepare you to work with a medical team to chart a path to eliminate that cancer. Part of that process involves establishing trust in the team of specialists who will care for them."

How do you build your inner strength? Talking things through with family or friends, a clergy member, or a therapist may aid you in finding the inner strength to cope with the new reality of having cancer. Dance, exercise, sports, board games, music, painting, and writing may assist you in accessing that strength at your core.

Treatment Guided By a Team

Your surgeon isn't acting alone. At the best medical centers, you are cared for by a team that consists of a breast surgeon, a medical oncologist, a radiation oncologist, a breast radiologist, and an experienced pathologist. Genetic counselors, integrative medicine specialists, pharmacologists, patient navigators, dietitians, nurses, nurse practitioners, physician assistants, social workers, and research scientists also frequently belong to or support such teams. Your primary care physician (PCP) is kept informed of your progress, and is an important part of long-term follow-up.

Because team members have training in many fields of science, we describe the medical treatment team as *multidisciplinary*. That is, experts from a wide range of scientific fields are working together to guide your treatment. Dr. Harness organized one of the first multidisciplinary breast centers in the United States.

When you see your surgeon outside the examining room reading messages on a handheld device or talking on the phone, you know that he or she is communicating with other specialists about your care. When your surgeon tells you that you were discussed at a meeting, you know your cancer was presented at a conference, where the facts of your case were weighed by many clinicians with unique perspectives on cancer. Individualized treatment plans emerge from such meetings, which influence the surgery and the other care that you receive.

Because surgery represents a critical step in treatment, it should fit into longer-term treatment planned by the multidisciplinary team. The presence of a team with long experience working together offers one way of ensuring the delivery of proper treatment that best addresses a woman's individual situation.

In some cases, the team recommends giving chemotherapy *before* the patient undergoes surgery.

Pre-Surgical Information Gathering

Good surgeons are sculptors. They think in three dimensions, and from the first time a surgeon examines you, he or she begins to form an idea of how you will look after surgery. The doctor imagines sculpting the breast, a breast mound, or the chest area to accommodate the outcome of your cancer surgery. The design develops as information about your cancer becomes available.

In the surgeon's mind, possibilities for removing your tumor range from a simple lumpectomy followed by artful reconstruction to a double mastectomy (removal of both breasts) with or without reconstruction. As more and more details about your cancer become available, the surgeon can successfully plan a procedure that will produce the best possible result. Before lifting the scalpel, the surgeon will have worked with you to determine the appropriate surgery for your breast cancer. Surgeons consider breast cancer type, size, and possible stage when selecting the kind of surgery a woman needs to treat a tumor.

Your genetic status may greatly impact action in the operating suite. A woman with breast cancer who carries the genes known as BRCA1 or BRCA2 may need a double mastectomy, a procedure that reduces a high risk of local recurrence. Afterward, many of these patients yearn for new breasts, a human factor that moves surgery across physical boundaries and into the domain of the human psyche.

When careful medical evaluation suggests that a woman needs a mastectomy, the surgeon ponders how to redesign the breast. Using his or her knowledge about plastic surgery, he or she chooses from an array of techniques to create the new breast mound. In making good choices that transform the breast area, the surgeon and a plastic surgeon address the needs of the whole woman.

The patient emerges from surgery with an improved health status, and she hopefully looks very good. After her surgical recovery, she also *feels good* about herself.

Identifying Breast Cancer

A woman's breast cancer journey begins when a doctor diagnoses a tumor in her breast.

There are three familiar paths that lead up to this diagnosis. A woman may feel a lump in her breast while showering or bathing or doing other routine activities; a health care provider may find a suspicious lump while performing a breast exam; or a routine mammogram may identify a suspicious area of the breast that appears to contain a mass or an abnormal group of microcalcifications. A doctor then takes a core biopsy; this involves removing a spaghetti-like sample of breast tissue that confirms the presence of a tumor.[1]

A tumor is an abnormal growth of tissue, and it can be benign or malignant. Of course, another term for malignant is *cancerous*. An identifiable tumor manifests as a collection or growth of abnormal tissue. An example of a common malignant breast tumor is an invasive ductal carcinoma (see Chapter 2).

Breast cancer represents a class of diseases so vast it seems like a constellation. This is why it's so important for a multidisplinary team to work on behalf of each patient. Scientists now believe breast cancer represents at least ten different diseases.[2]

Determining the type of tumor you have and identifying its characteristics can take time. Obtaining important information from other studies may take even more time.

There are multiple diagnostic tools that help determine cancer status:

- An ultrasound and a breast MRI will reveal the shape and size of the tumor. If an MRI is done, it may also identify whether more than one tumor exists in the diagnosed breast, and whether the other breast is affected; it can also identify lymph nodes that appear abnormal.

- If necessary, PET/CT (positron emission tomography/computed tomography) scanning provides information about the possible spread of the cancer to other areas of the body, such as the bones.

- A chest x-ray provides information about the heart and lungs.

As mentioned above, the core biopsy is one of the first ways to make a definitive diagnosis after a suspicious lump is found. Clinicians examine a cylinder of breast tissue to obtain information about the *histology* of a cancer. They insert a needle into the breast to obtain the required core of tissue. Material collected with such biopsies permits clinicians to identify tumor type and *tumor markers* (see below) in a breast cancer.

These tests allow doctors to begin to "fingerprint" a woman's cancer—that is, to identify its unique characteristics. This

The pathologist grades the tumor based on the size of its cells and how uniform they are; how fast tumor cells are dividing; and the percentage of tube-like structures that exist in the tumor.

fingerprint emerges from the results of the core biopsy and imaging studies. Aspects of the fingerprint tell the treatment team whether the tumor is *in situ* or *invasive,* and whether it is *ductal* or *lobular,* and help identify the *grade* of the tumor, an indication of its aggressiveness. The fingerprint also provides information about the tumor's *markers.*

Markers reveal the aggressiveness of a tumor, a factor of great importance to the treatment team. Among the markers used to gather information about a tumor are:

- Estrogen receptor status, positive or negative.

- Progesterone receptor status, positive or negative.

- HER-2/neu status, positive or negative.

- Ki-67 status

The identification of any of these markers in a woman's tumor has major implications for the type of treatment she receives. Women with hormone receptor positive status get long-term drug treatment designed to block estrogen and to help prevent cancer recurrence. One tumor marker reveals if a breast cancer is HER-2-neu positive, indicating a more aggressive type of breast cancer. The Ki-67 marker provides information about how rapidly breast cancer cells are dividing and forming new cancer cells.

Initial fingerprinting tells us where we are within the constellation and helps us assess how to treat a woman's breast cancer.

During this fingerprinting stage—and during the treatment itself—your doctor will be assisted by a team of specialists who have different and complementary skills.

Radiologists formally read the medical "pictures" of your tumor that will be used by all members of the treatment team. (Doctors who are most adept at reading such pictures usually complete programs that provide special training in breast imaging.)

The skills of the radiologist help prepare the surgeon to eradicate the tumor growing in your breast. The radiologist's work informs the surgeon of the tumor's shape, size, and location. If there is more than one tumor in the breast (or if a tumor or tumors exist in the other breast), the radiologist confirms its presence with a core biopsy.

The pathologist is another important member of your breast cancer treatment team. He or she takes the role of a fingerprint specialist, establishing the identity of the criminal that has invaded your body, and identifying the risks the thug poses for you. Pathologists know if the criminal is aggressive or mild-mannered. They learn this by studying tissue to obtain clues about the invader and about the environment the thug has entered.

In their minds, pathologists carry images of the types of cancer cells and compare them to the images they see on slides made with your own tissue. With these, they identify the bad actors in the breast. The pathologist not only identifies the criminal (cancer type) that has invaded your body, but also describes it in detail. This specialist predicts how bad the criminal is (from cell type, grade, and markers), which may provide insight into the possible course the criminal's behavior may take.

The skills of a pathologist greatly enhance the work of your treatment team because the highly variable nature of the biology of breast tumors influences how treatment plans are personalized.

The pathologist grades the tumor based on the size of its cells and how uniform they are; how fast tumor cells are dividing; and the percentage of tube-like structures that exist in the tumor. Scoring is often done with the modified Scarff-Bloom-Richardson grading system.

The grade the pathologist assigns to the tumor, along with the report of its markers, establishes the degree of criminality of the invader in the body.

The information the pathologist gathers establishes whether treatment with anti-estrogen hormone therapy, chemotherapy, or targeted therapy can effectively combat your cancer. As such, it defines which of these treatments should be used—and using all three may be an option.

Well-differentiated tumors—those with fairly uniform cells—grow slowly. Those with wild differences in the cells—i.e., poorly differentiated tumors—grow quickly and are more dangerous.

A fingerprint that identifies a high-grade tumor indicates an aggressive, more rapidly growing cancer. It's an offender to take seriously and stop. Tumors labeled as *ductal carcinoma in situ* usually measure as low or intermediate grade cancers. When they've progressed to high grade, however, they're ugly and mean.

Invasive cancers, by definition, escape from the milk ducts and may show up as well-differentiated, moderately differentiated, or poorly differentiated tumors.

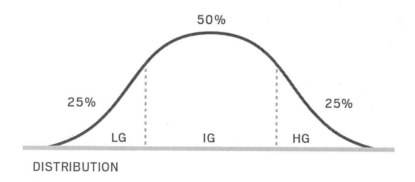

When illustrated on a bell curve (a chart that plots frequency distribution), the growth rates of most tumors are slow. On this curve, most tumors fall into intermediate grades and are charted in the middle of the curve.

Slow-growing tumors show up on the left side of the chart, aggressive tumors on the right, reflecting the continuum of aggressiveness. As treatment teams work to accurately diagnose tumors and come up with individualized treatment plans, this tumor distribution phenomenon works in women's favor. Most tumors do not grow very quickly.

Endnotes

1. Patients may be more comfortable during a biopsy if they take Tylenol for several days before undergoing a biopsy. Patients should ask for and obtain all reports and all patient procedure instructions.

2. Curtis C, et al. The genomic and transcriptomic architecture of 2000 breast tumors. Nature [serial online] 2012; Apr 18.

Chapter 2

Treatment Planning: A Journey of Discovery

Eliminating breast cancer from the human body presents doctors and patients with a challenge. Together, they undertake a journey to discover possibilities for healing. By examining the tumor, they learn more about the disease the woman confronts.

This cancer journey often reveals the context in which the disease arose. As truths reveal themselves, doctors gain insights about their patients. A woman who has been diagnosed with breast cancer may grapple with her new identity as a person with breast cancer while refusing to allow cancer to define her.

Doctors obtain information about the tumor. Patients learn more about their bodies and how to take care of them. The information obtained offers a tool of liberation: for doctors, it shapes the way they help women resist the disease; for women, it helps contain their fear of the disease.

Most women realize their breasts can feed children, enchant lovers, and form an aspect of their female figure. What's inside the breasts is another matter, however, and many women don't give it much thought.

As an organ, the human breast inspires awe. Underneath a beautiful envelope of skin, the female breast contains a complex anatomy. Fat deposits help create the spongy feel of a breast.[1] A system of structures called *lobules* allows the breast to secrete milk. Each breast also contains multiple milk ducts. Lobules exist at the beginning of these ducts. At the crest of the breast, a nipple provides a mechanism for extracting milk. Its engineering is marvelous—structures in the areola can lubricate the nipple, helping a mother endure the dryness and the soreness that sometimes goes with the sharp nips of a feeding baby.

Scientists believe breast cancer arises in special tissue in the breast called terminal ductal lobular units (TDLUs). A tumor begins against the background of a changing environment in the breast, a domain influenced by the stages of a woman's life and her age. Women over 50, who usually don't use their breasts to produce milk and who may no longer regularly menstruate, are more likely to get breast cancer than younger women.[2]

Cancer begins when a cell develops a mutation in an important area of its DNA, and this change alters the potential behavior of the cell. In the breast, it theoretically flourishes if it finds a domain that promotes and puts up with mutated cells. The disease can continuously change, and malignant cells can evolve.[3]

Physicians look for four general types of breast cancer. Two types of cancer remain contained in the ducts and lobules of the breast. Doctors refer to these types of tumors as noninvasive, or *in situ*.

Physicians look for four general types of breast cancer. Two types of cancer remain contained in the ducts and lobules of the breast. Doctors refer to these types of tumors as noninvasive, or in situ.

1. *Ductal carcinoma in situ* (DCIS) arises in *ducts* and remains there.

2. *Lobular carcinoma in situ* (LCIS) starts in the *lobules* and remains there.

LCIS is usually not a cancer, but a precancerous marker lesion that reveals an increased future risk of breast cancer. DCIS is cancerous. Information about treatment of ductal carcinomas can be found in Chapter 5.

The other two types of cancer escape the ducts or lobules and invade the surrounding breast tissue. Doctors refer to these types of tumors as *invasive*.

3. *Invasive lobular carcinoma* (also called *infiltrating lobular carcinoma*) escapes the lobule.

4. *Invasive ductal carcinoma* (also called *infiltrating ductal carcinoma*) moves outside the duct.

An invasive cancer can shed malignant cells that are capable of circulating elsewhere in the body through the venous system (the veins) and the lymphatic (lymph) system. Once these cancer cells begin circulating in the body, they can create *micrometastasis*, a clustering of cells so small that no current imaging technology can identify it. These potential micrometastasis are the reason that patients with invasive breast cancers require treatment of the whole body (systemic therapy—see Chapter 7).

A physician treating a woman who has breast cancer works to determine the extent of the disease she faces. Doctors measure the extent by describing the cancer's stage. The medical staging system provides a consistent way of talking about breast cancer, as well as other types of cancers. Among other things, the stage helps predict survival. A staging system, referred to as the TNM approach, provides information on the tumor (tumor = T), including size and extent (classified Tis to 4); the lymph nodes (nodes = N), including number, character, and location (often classified 0 to 3); and metastasis (metastasis = M), or proof of spread to other organs (0 or 1, none or spread).

TNM Stages for Breast Cancer

Stage	T	N	M
Stage 0	Tis	N0	M0
Stage I	T1	N0	M0
Stage IIA	T0 T1 T2	N1 N1 N0	M0 M0 M0
Stage IIB	T2 T3	N1 N0	M0 M0
Stage IIIA	T0-2 T3	N2 N1-2	M0 M0
Stage IIIB	T4	N0-2	M0
Stage IIIC	Any T	N3	M0
Stage IV	Any T	Any N	M1

Source: American Cancer Society

Stage 0 includes in situ cancers, and the tumor is Tis (Tis, N0, M0).

Stage I and even Stage II cancers often represent an early form of breast cancer. A minimally invasive cancer might measure as a T1, have no cancerous lymph nodes (N0), and show no evidence of spread to other organs (M0), resulting in a T1, N0, M0 tumor. A locally advanced tumor (Stage III) might be classified as a T3, N2, M0.

Using staging information, doctors can describe patients who share similar characteristics, which helps predict outcomes and allows patients to be matched to treatment strategies based on their stage and risk.

Stage I cancers measure as small (2 centimeters or smaller, some .79 inches), with no evidence of spread to lymph nodes or other sites. Tumors that measure over 2 centimeters or that have spread to lymph nodes fall into Stage II or III. Breast cancers that have spread to other areas of the body are described as Stage IV.[4]

In recent years, national medical review panels have added subcategories to the stages to better describe breast cancer. These panels are currently struggling to reconcile a gap between emerging knowledge about the biology of breast cancer and how this new information should reshape the established staging system and its application to clinical practice. Fueling this struggle are rapidly evolving molecular descriptions of breast cancer that define subgroups of the disease that respond differently to treatment and give women different chances for survival. These developments suggest that the TNM system alone may not determine treatment decisions now and in the future.

Staging is not necessarily static. Each time a woman is staged for her breast cancer, the evaluation represents a "still life" view of a disease known to show dynamic changes over time.[5]

Treatment Pathways

Women with different types of cancer have different journeys to recovery. Distinct pathways exist for the treatment of *in situ* cancer and *invasive* cancer. These pathways can be likened to a trail with many branches. As doctors track the cancer, they advise women to take appropriate branches along the journey.

Noninvasive Cancer

For a woman with ductal carcinoma in situ (DCIS), a surgeon may perform a lumpectomy (partial mastectomy) or a mastectomy, depending on the size and grade of the tumor. Radiation therapy may also be needed after lumpectomy, but not always.

Theoretically, mastectomy cures DCIS because this tumor does not invade the breast. There are exceptions to this rule, but in general, women with DCIS who choose mastectomy will need no systemic therapy, including chemotherapy or anti-hormonal therapy. The primary role of anti-estrogen (anti-hormonal) medication in DCIS patients who undergo mastectomy is for its ability to lower the risk of subsequent cancer in the woman's remaining breast.

A woman with lobular carcinoma in situ (LCIS) may simply be monitored by doctors for signs of a later possible cancer; surgery is usually not recommended. LCIS is generally viewed as a marker lesion that increases the lifetime risk of developing breast cancer. Surgeons typically find LCIS when performing a breast biopsy for some other reason.[6]

Invasive Cancer

With invasive breast cancer, malignant cells invade the breast and circulate through the body. Tumors can then grow in other organs, threatening the woman's life.

Modern tools help physicians track down the location of breast cancers, in and outside the breast. Ultrasound is one of those tools. Ultrasound machines utilize high-frequency sound waves to view structures below the skin in the breast and other organs. They produce images of tumors and normal organs.

Two major surgical pathways exist to eradicate invasive cancer found in the breast.

Surgeons can perform breast-conserving surgery (lumpectomy) for many smaller invasive breast cancers, although mastectomy is also an option.

When the tumor is large or aggressive, a surgeon will generally perform a mastectomy, unless chemotherapy or anti-hormonal therapy can shrink the tumor first. Large or aggressive tumors may require chemotherapy or anti-hormonal therapy prior to surgery. This treatment approach is known as *neoadjuvant* therapy.

Women with invasive cancers who opt for lumpectomy rather than mastectomy will likely need *adjunctive* (post-surgery) radiation therapy. Treatment regimens may be altered based on staging information, but the TNM staging system alone should not determine adjuvant therapy; important molecular tests now augment the system.

Tools

Physicians use an important set of tools to identify cancer in the body. They select helpful tools and employ different combinations of the tools, depending on the woman being diagnosed.

Mammography

Mammography produces an image of the breast using x-rays. The image shows the structures of the breast and allows a radiologist to look at unusual areas of the breast, especially suspicious regions.

Images obtained via mammography can identify lesions as small as 0.2 centimeter (0.08 inch), whereas a tumor must often grow to 1 centimeter (0.4 inch) before a doctor can feel it.

Mammograms only take images of parts of the breast that project outward. Plates used for the exam are positioned underneath or on the sides of the breast, and getting an accurate picture of a large breast is easier than obtaining a picture of a small one.

Some mammograms screen for cancer, while others help diagnose cancer. Diagnostic mammograms may be obtained to look for breast cancer after the discovery of a lump or other signs or symptoms. For example, your doctor may send you for a mammogram if your breasts are lumpy and a prominent lump is found. Other reasons to look for breast cancer may include breast pain, thickening of the breast skin, nipple discharge, nipple retraction, or a change in breast size or shape.

During this test, diagnostic mammograms show the breast from several angles. A technician may opt to magnify an area to provide a detailed picture that can assist a radiologist in making a correct diagnosis of a suspicious site.

If a lump shows up as jagged on a mammogram, it's a sign that further tests are needed. That's because as cancers grow, they position themselves between normal cells, or "infiltrate," and produce irregular, jagged edges. This is often how invasive breast cancers look on mammograms. The next test would be an ultrasound examination of the suspicious area seen on the mammogram.

All conventional mammograms produce a two-dimensional image of a three-dimensional organ. Less dense tissue may appear as gray or black. Areas that are denser, including cancers, show up brighter. The breast tissue of young women may be very dense and show up as white on mammograms. For that reason, mammograms are less sensitive in showing cancers in young women as reliably as in older women. Older women usually have more fat in their breasts, making it easier for mammograms to identify tumors.

Modern mammography devices produce digital images that physicians can view on a computer screen. These images can be manipulated with software, magnified and contrast-adjusted to reveal important aspects of a tumor, including small differences in nearby tissues. Emerging technology now provides 3-D mammograms that show the breast in three dimensions. In such images, the breast is imaged in slices.

Radiologists typically diagnose ductal carcinoma in situ (DCIS) with mammograms, through the identification of an area of branching microcalcifications (calcium deposits) that vary in size and shape. DCIS can also present as a mass on a mammogram or on a physical examination.

No single imaging technology produces perfect results. The three main technologies—mammography, ultrasound, and MRI—are complementary to each other. Thus, a "negative" diagnostic mammogram for a woman with a suspicious lump also requires a negative ultrasound and/or MRI before the results are truly negative.

No single imaging technology produces perfect results. The three main technologies—mammography, ultrasound, and MRI—are complementary to each other. Thus, a "negative" diagnostic mammogram for a woman with a suspicious lump also requires a negative ultrasound and/or MRI before the results are truly negative.

Ultrasound

High-frequency sound waves help reveal details inside the breast. This ultrasound technology often provides important information in cases of invasive cancer, but there's a limit to what this technology can do.

Many women develop lumpy areas in their breasts, and most of them do not have cancer. But physicians want to examine suspicious regions to rule out malignancy. With ultrasound, surgeons and radiologists can determine whether a lumpy area of the breast is something to worry about or something to discount. Ultrasound also helps your physician to learn whether a mass in your breast formed as a solid or as a cyst, or if it shows characteristics common to tumors.

Ultrasound helps physicians to characterize what a mass looks like. Certain characteristics that show up on an ultrasound exam indicate whether a tumor is benign, and others tell whether a mass may be malignant. When a breast surgeon palpates the breast, they rely on their fingers to do certain things. Ultrasound extends their fingers by helping them look beneath the skin.

Ultrasound also guides biopsies, enabling a clinician to see a needle as he or she inserts it to drain (aspirate) a cyst or to do a core biopsy of an area. During surgery, ultrasound assists the surgeon in performing important procedures that locate tumors. For these reasons, this technology provides an important diagnostic and adjunctive tool.

Breast MRI

An imaging strategy known as breast MRI plays a very important role in the evaluation of newly diagnosed

> *MRI may be most helpful in women with dense breasts.*

patients with breast cancer, although not all specialists agree on this point. MRI employs magnets to produce images of tissue in the breast. The main reasons to obtain a breast MRI are:

- To look for disease in other areas of the breast

- To determine the extent of the cancer

- To look for involvement of lymph nodes in the region of the breast.[7]

Women with in situ and invasive cancer may benefit from MRI. MRI may find cancers that fail to show up on mammograms or on ultrasound studies. For this reason, a breast MRI may identify additional invasive and noninvasive tumors in the affected breast and in the opposite breast.

MRI may be most helpful in women with dense breasts. Dense breast tissue shows up as white on imaging studies, and most breast cancers also show up as white. If you have white (dense breast tissue) on white (breast cancer), the cancer may be invisible on a mammogram but visible on an MRI or ultrasound study.

Physicians often order breast MRI after obtaining digital mammograms and ultrasound studies and after establishing a patient's diagnosis of breast cancer.[8] Most insurance companies refuse to pay for an MRI of the breasts unless a biopsy establishes a diagnosis of cancer or the patient is known to be BRCA 1 or BRCA 2 gene positive.

What comes next depends on the results of the breast MRI. Among other things, breast MRI may help to determine whether cancer exists in the nipple-areola area of the breast. About 15 percent of the time, additional biopsies may be needed after obtaining a breast MRI for a woman with non-invasive or invasive breast cancer. If a second or third suspicious area shows up on the MRI, a physician may also order a "second look" ultrasound to see if a tumor is in the area, as well as additional biopsies. If nothing shows up on a second-look ultrasound, radiologists may conduct an MRI-guided biopsy to define the abnormal area.

For invasive cancers, breast MRI may also help to determine whether lymph nodes inside the chest, in the armpit (axillary) area, and in the base of the neck contain observable cancer. If they do, clinicians may then conduct an ultrasound-guided biopsy to further investigate the possible spread of the patient's cancer to the lymph nodes. All this information helps the multidisciplinary team determine what to do for the patient.

Critics of breast MRI argue that these imaging studies find very small tumors that could be eradicated with radiation therapy rather than surgery. Detection of some of these tumors, along with false-positive results, they say, leads to unnecessary biopsies and surgery.

Breast MRIs also assist in detecting recurrence in patients originally treated for locally advanced (Stage III) invasive breast cancers. This is true for those with Stage III cancers who opted for mastectomy with or without breast reconstruction. Insurers typically pay for breast MRIs for such patients.

Continuing use of MRI provides more insight into when it can be most helpful. A German study involving 1,500 patients showed that surgeons changed their treatment strategy in 12 to 13 percent of cases when they obtained preoperative MRIs. The greatest shift came in the treatment of patients with invasive lobular carcinoma. During surgery, surgeons often appropriately excised more breast tissue in these patients. German national guidelines now recommend obtaining a preoperative breast MRI in patients with invasive lobular carcinoma verified by examining tissue under a microscope.[9]

For women with BRCA 1 and BRCA 2 genes, breast MRI becomes part of the annual screening process. Coverage for annual breast MRIs is also extended for patients with a lifetime risk of breast cancer greater than 22 to 23 percent.

Sampling Lymph Nodes

Knowing the status of lymph nodes helps women and their doctors measure the aggressiveness of the tumor a woman is confronting.

In cases of invasive cancer, scientists know that cancer cells can travel through the lymphatic channels that go to lymph nodes and begin growing in the nodes. These channels are like a Route 66 for cancer cells. The lymph system represents one of the first drainage areas from the breast, typically in the axilla, or armpit. To cancer cells, the place under your arm is like a highway rest stop along the route. So it's one of the areas from which the surgeon can take tissue biopsies to see if a cancerous tumor has spread.

Lymph nodes are part of our defense system. They are our local neighborhood warriors. When you have an infection arising from a bad tooth, the lymph nodes in the neck swell up because the nodes are producing antibodies to help fight the infection. But when breast cancer arises, as malignant cells invade the body and circulate, surgeons often need to remove lymph nodes that contain cancer. (There are exceptions.)

Before surgery, it is possible to sample lymph nodes using a technique known as ultrasound-guided needle biopsy. Such biopsies are also frequently done during surgery. This is called *sentinel node biopsy* (SNB). A negative SNB means the surgeon can avoid removing any additional axillary lymph nodes.

Determining Menopausal Status and Treatment

Learning the menopausal status of a woman with breast cancer provides important information. Age, menstrual history, and blood tests usually ordered by medical oncologists determine menopausal status.

Doctors refer to women as either premenopausal, perimenopausal, or postmenopausal. Their menopausal status influences the choice of any anti-estrogen medication prescribed to them. Some women receive anti-estrogen medication prior to surgery in an attempt to shrink their tumors, and continue to take it after surgery.

Medical oncologists may prescribe chemotherapy for pre-, peri-, and postmenopausal patients with invasive cancer. Genomic tests can also be used to determine the need for chemotherapy (see Chapter 7).

Mapping the Cancer Journey

Taken together, information obtained from patient histories, core biopsies, digital mammograms, ultrasound, breast MRI, and lymph node sampling prepares a woman to make a decision about the type of surgery she wants to undergo for breast cancer: breast-conserving lumpectomy or mastectomy.

Data obtained from imaging and other diagnostic studies helps the multidisciplinary team begin sketching out a map for use on the patient's cancer journey. Once the treatment team establishes a diagnosis, the map of the patient's cancer journey begins to show more detail. The extent of disease is determined, options are discussed with the patient and her family, and the journey begins in earnest. A personalized treatment plan is developed that outlines the beginning, middle, and lifelong points on the journey. Then the plan is executed, and actions for long-term follow-up are formulated.

While these maps are different for every woman, there are common themes. Women with small cancers, which are often detected during mammogram screenings, may decide to undergo lumpectomy and radiation therapy procedures that control the cancerous tumor and the area surrounding it. Those with invasive cancer get systemic therapy designed to rid the whole body of cancer (these therapies can include chemotherapy, anti-hormonal therapy, and targeted therapy).

On such maps, the work of a medical oncologist more and more frequently intersects with that of the surgeon. The treatment known as neoadjuvant therapy provides an example of a strategy that helps some women. Neoadjuvant (before surgery) therapy generally takes four to six months to complete. Medical oncologists administer the chemotherapy or anti-hormonal therapy that comprise this therapy.[10,11,12]

Neoadjuvant therapy is one approach that treats the whole body, providing systemic treatment to help eradicate cancer throughout the body. Neoadjuvant therapy may also reduce the extent of surgery required to provide treatment of the primary tumor and the area surrounding the tumor.[8,13]

Oncologists also use clinical descriptions for breast cancer, with major categories of invasive breast cancer described as:

- Early stage invasive breast cancer (Stages I and II), usually involving tumors smaller than five centimeters in diameter, with or without spread to specific lymph nodes.

- Locally advanced breast cancer, which involves a broad range of tumors. Malignancies may be large, with spread to lymph nodes but without metastasis to other organs.

- Inflammatory breast cancer, a rare and aggressive cancer often confused with an infection of the breast. A physician frequently finds no mass in the breast but discovers a pink or extremely red area of the breast that feels warm to the touch.

Endnotes

1. Love, S, Lindsey, K., *Dr. Susan Love's Breast Book*. 5th ed. Boston: Da Capo Press, 2010, 890

2. Ibid.

3. Ibid.

4. Ibid.

5. Ibid.

6. Singletary, SE, Robb GL, Hortobagyi GN. Advanced Therapy of Disease. 2nd ed. Beijing, China: PMPH; 2004.

7. Sardanelli F. Overview of the role of pre-operative breast MRI in the absence of evidence on patient outcomes. Breast 2010; 19(1):3–6.

8. In premenopausal women, MRIs should be taken within the first two weeks of a menstrual cycle.

9. Fischer, U. Practical MR Mammography: High Resolution MRI of the Breast. 2nd ed. Stuttgart, Germany: Thieme; 2012.

10. van Rijk, MC. Sentinel node biopsy before neoadjuvant chemotherapy spares breast cancer patients axillary lymph node dissection. Ann Surg Oncol 2006; 13(4): 475–9

11. Mittendorf, E, et al. Validation of a novel staging system for disease-specific survival in patients with breast cancer treated with neoadjuvant chemotherapy. J Clin Oncol 2011; 29(15): 1956–62

12. Mittendorf EA, et al. Impact of chemotherapy sequencing on local-regional failure risk in breast cancer patients undergoing breast-conserving therapy.

13. Adjuvant and Neoadjuvant Therapy for Breast Cancer. Available at cancer.gov/cancertopics/factsheet/Therapy/adjuvant-breast. Accessed Sept 22, 2013.

Chapter 3

Lumpectomy or Mastectomy: Issues in Decision Making

All the information collected about a patient and her cancer helps determine the type of surgery the surgeon ultimately recommends. The process of gathering the facts can easily take days or a few weeks if genetic and other testing is needed. Once the information is analyzed, the vision for the future of your breast becomes clearer.

Your surgeon determines what procedures he or she can use to help you. There are several types of procedures to remove breast cancer from the body or defend against it.

They include:

Lumpectomy. In this surgery, also known as breast-conserving surgery, a cancerous lump is removed from the breast, along with a rim of normal breast tissue around it

Mastectomy. In this surgery, the breast is removed. Based on the gathered information, surgeons can use different techniques for this type of surgery.

- A skin-sparing mastectomy is a removal of the breast that preserves a large amount of skin for use in reconstruction.

- A *nipple-sparing mastectomy* is a removal of the breast that preserves the skin, the areola, and the nipple in cases in which the tumor does not involve the nipple or the areola.

- Sentinel lymph node biopsy is the removal of the sentinel lymph nodes, the first ones to collect lymphatic drainage from the breast.

- A total mastectomy is the removal of only the breast.

- A modified radical mastectomy is the removal of the breast and lymph nodes in the armpit (axilla).

- A *prophylactic mastectomy* (or *preventive mastectomy*) is the removal of one or both breasts to reduce the risk of developing breast cancer.

Surgeons are often able to give their patients a choice between lumpectomy and mastectomy. Many patients struggle with this decision. Patients need to know that in properly selected cases of breast cancer, clinical trials show no difference in long-term survival in patients who choose breast conservation—that is, a lumpectomy—rather than mastectomy. Long-term survival depends on the biology of the cancer and on the individual's situation.

Surgeons understand that women find it difficult to make choices about surgery. Patients face a dilemma. Everything the surgeon recommends offers benefits and involves a downside. Fortunately, with lumpectomy, a patient keeps her breast. Unfortunately, a small chance arises each year that the cancer can return to the breast the surgeon saved. The lifetime risk is roughly 8 to 12 percent in properly selected patients.

Women who opt for breast conservation also usually need some type of radiation therapy, such as partial breast radiation therapy or full breast radiation therapy.

With mastectomy, most women don't need radiation therapy. Over the remaining years of a woman's life, only a small chance exists of a cancer recurring at a mastectomy site.

Nationally, more and more women now choose mastectomy. They make this choice for many reasons. The fear of a recurrence of cancer in the breast ranks at the top, not surprisingly. Avoiding radiation therapy comes in second. The fact that reconstruction surgery techniques have evolved and improved over time also greatly influences patients' decisions—quite simply, surgeons can create better, more natural looking breasts now than they could in the past.

For women who are deciding between lumpectomy and mastectomy, we recommend that they get their care at centers that frequently do breast conservation and also offer high-end reconstruction after mastectomy.

As you make your decision about which surgery to undergo, take time for yourself. You're experiencing a life-altering event.

How much your cancer diagnosis will alter your life is yet to be defined, but one thing is certain: making good decisions will be important. You can help yourself by creating an environment that supports careful thought and reflection. Part of that process involves connecting with your heart.

The late psychologist Joan Erikson, who was married to the famed developmental psychologist and psychoanalyst Erik Erikson, saw decision-making as akin to pulling threads while weaving a tapestry. Some answers in life come from the heart, she told a friend. "It's about give and take, pulling and tugging, working it through, like … weavings."[1]

As you discover how you feel about the choices you are considering for surgery, honor yourself and listen to your heart. There are practical ways to do so: Get out in nature. Prepare meals using fresh foods, for a diet helpful to your heart. Use moderate exercise to reduce inflammation in your body. Play lyrical music. Drink tea. Eat only good fats and foods low in fats (and after treatment ends, reduce your weight to a normal range). Consult a dentist with expertise in preventing problems in the mouth. If you live in a big city and drive to and from work, travel at non-peak hours to reduce your stress.

Ask your surgeon to refer you to an integrative medicine specialist who can advise you on preparing your body for the demanding medical journey ahead. Use daily readings of positive affirmations to focus your intention on healing, to create calm, and to engender faith. Work to limit stressors in your life. Talk with a supportive friend, strive for emotional balance, and prepare to take action.

Keeping a daily journal puts you in touch with your thoughts and feelings. We suggest that you write down how you feel about the choice you are trying to make. In the end, no perfect answers ever emerge. Each choice extends benefits; each choice exacts sacrifices. Make what you feel is the right decision for you.

The act of making a decision about surgery creates a shift in your attitude toward your cancer, from fear to empowerment. You're taking an action that gets events moving. "Many of us would just as soon have our choices made for us," a Jungian analyst told American writer Joan Anderson, "but the heroine, when at a juncture, makes her own choice."[2]

> *Women who experience a complete pathological response to neoadjuvant therapy—meaning the tissue removed during their surgery is free of active cancer cells—may have a better prognosis than other women with the same stage and type of cancer.*

Neoadjuvant Therapy

One of your choices may involve use of a treatment known as neoadjuvant therapy. This treatment may lower the burden of the cancer in your breast and/or lymph nodes. It may even "downstage" your cancer, depending on the results. (Women who experience a complete pathological response to neoadjuvant therapy—meaning the tissue removed during their surgery is free of active cancer cells—may have a better prognosis than other women with the same stage and type of cancer.) Neoadjuvant therapy may do far more than help some women make decisions about surgery; depending on the strength of your response to this therapy, it may help change the course of your treatment. It also begins the process of treating your whole body, an approach needed to treat all invasive cancers.

Neoadjuvant chemotherapy reduces the size of tumors with drugs or anti-hormonal therapy *before* a patient goes into surgery. This potentially helps some women avoid mastectomy, even those with advanced breast cancers. That is, surgery in breasts can sometimes be minimized and breasts saved.[3,4,5]

Ask your doctor whether this therapy would help you.

Genetic Testing and Counseling

If a woman is 50 or younger when she first develops breast cancer, or if she has close relatives (mother, sisters, aunts, father, uncles, cousins) with a history of breast or ovarian cancer, genetic counseling and testing is indicated.

Women who undergo testing will learn whether they carry the breast cancer susceptibility genes BRCA1 and BRCA2. They use the information obtained to decide whether to receive breast-conserving surgery or mastectomy. If they carry either gene, they face a high risk of breast cancer recurrence following lumpectomy and radiation; thus many women who test positive for either gene opt for mastectomy. Those who do not are closely monitored with the goal of rapidly detecting any breast cancer that does develop.

Mastectomy Choices

For patients who ultimately undergo mastectomy, reconstruction can produce attractive breasts. Because of surgical advances, your nipple may even be saved.[6] In the past, surgeons discarded the nipple and the pigmented area around it called the areola when they performed a skin-sparing mastectomy.

That procedure prepares the mastectomy site for reconstruction, using a tissue expander or tissue from other parts of the body. Tissue expanders are thick, breast-shaped balloons; they are similar to breast implants, but when they're first inserted under or on top of the chest muscles (the *pectoralis major*) after a mastectomy, they're fairly flat. In a series of sessions during the first stage of reconstructive surgery, plastic surgeons fill an expander with fluid. This expansion reshapes the chest area and creates the appearance of a new breast.

Later, in the second stage of reconstruction, a plastic surgeon replaces the temporary expander with a permanent implant, or replaces it with tissue taken from other areas of the patient's body.

Today, many women keep their nipples after a mastectomy. In the past, nipples were not saved due to three concerns:

1. Maintaining an adequate blood supply to the nipple and areola during surgery

2. The possibility of a cancer coming back at the nipple or areola

3. The potential presence of cancer in the nipple at the time of surgery.[7,8]

If you're considering nipple-sparing mastectomy, turn to surgeons experienced with the technique. Go to a center with a multidisciplinary team that fully images the breast. Get digital mammograms, ultrasound, and a breast MRI that shows what's in the breast and that the nipple and areola are not affected by the cancer.

Reconstructions are usually done in stages. So ensure that your center uses plastic surgeons who are capable of performing first- and second-stage breast reconstructions. Such services are usually provided at a facility that employs advanced treatments. My own center has performed over 600 nipple-sparing mastectomies. Although women lose sensation with this surgery, they report being very, very happy with the cosmetic result.

Sparing a nipple is not always an option, but plastic surgeons can often shape a new one, as will be discussed in Chapters 5 and 6.

1. Anderson J. *A Year By the Sea*. New York, NY: Broadway Books; 1999: 97–98, 100, 116–117.

2. Ibid.

3. van Rijk, MC. Sentinel node biopsy before neoadjuvant chemotherapy spares breast cancer patients axillary lymph node dissection. Ann Surg Oncol 2006; 13(4):

4. Mittendorf, E, et al. Validation of a novel staging system for disease-specific survival in patients with breast cancer treated with neoadjuvant chemotherapy. J Clin Oncol 2011; 29(15): 1956–62

5. Cruz CS, et al. Magnetic resonance imaging in breast cancer treated with neoadjuvant chemotherapy: Radiologic-pathologic correlation of the response and disease-free survival depending on molecular subtype. Radiologia 2013 Jan 4. pii: S0033-8338(12)00272-X. doi: 10.1016/j.rx.2012.10.004.

6. Spears S., et al. Nipple-sparing mastectomy for prophylactic and therapeutic indications. Plast Reconstr Surg 2011; 128(5): 1005–1014.

7. Harness, JK, Vetter, TS, Salibian, AH. Areola and nipple-areola-sparing mastectomy for breast cancer treatment and risk reduction: Report of an initial experience in a community hospital setting. Ann Surg Oncol 2011: 18: 917–922

8. Salibian, AH, Harness, JK, Mowlds, DS. Inframmary approach to nipple-areola-sparing mastectomy. Plast Reconstr Surg 2013; 132(5):700e–708e.

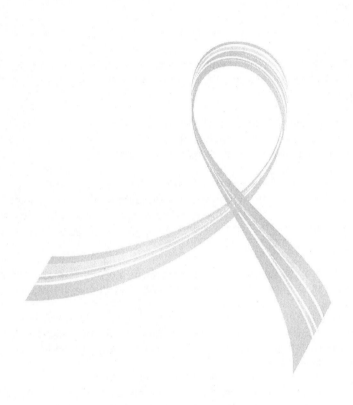

Chapter 4

Unseen Guides: The Roles of Pathologists and Radiation Oncologists

When you go into surgery, important members of the surgical team come with you. You will seldom see these physicians, but it is important to know what they do. The roles of the pathologist and radiation oncologist are covered here.

Breast Cancer Pathologist

Pathologists are important guides along your cancer journey. Although you don't know they're with you, they make a profound contribution to your care and greatly influence the options that mark the turning points on your cancer journey.

Pathologists train to dissect and analyze tissue and blood removed from the body. They determine whether these substances contain cancer. During surgery to remove a breast tumor, these doctors work with the surgeon to examine the tumor excised from the body.

Pathologists also determine whether cancer exists in the lymph nodes, which may also be examined during or after surgery. They use *sentinel node biopsy* (SNB) to do so. The sentinel lymph nodes, the first ones to collect lymphatic drainage from the breast, are removed and examined. The tissue is thinly sliced, put on small glass slides, stained with color, and put under a microscope.

"Every day I go into the operating room, a pathologist is available," Dr. Harness says. "I ask the pathologist to examine a cancer during surgery to see whether I've gotten clear margins, which means the edges of the cancer I removed are tumor free."

The work of the pathologist also further describes more features of the woman's tumor. "While I'm operating, the pathologist may perform frozen sections on lymph nodes, which allow rapid analysis of this tissue. These frozen sections of the tissue are examined under a microscope, and they let me know whether or not the nodes contain cancer. Knowledge gained from the work of the pathologist often helps avoid taking the patient in for additional surgeries."

Not every woman gets an SNB, which examines the first lymph nodes where a tumor drains. Some get fine needle aspirations or core biopsies on enlarged lymph nodes prior to surgery, and these provide information on the cancer status of the lymph nodes. Detecting cancer in these nodes helps surgeons remove the nodes that are at highest risk of containing cancer cells during breast cancer surgery. Malignant cells often invade nodes in the axilla (armpit). If a sentinel node is positive, other lymph nodes located beyond it may contain cancer.

Performing a Sentinel Node Biopsy

A surgeon locates a sentinel node by using a radioactive tracer, a blue dye, or both. The doctor injects the tracer and/or blue dye in one of several possible locations in the breast to discover where the cancer cells would travel. Finding the route reveals which of the first few lymph nodes (if any) are likely to test positive for cancer.

Invasive Breast Cancer

Several situations call for the use of SNB. If a patient is diagnosed with an invasive breast cancer by core biopsy, sentinel lymph node biopsy can help "stage" the patient, enabling the doctor to learn whether the cancer has gone from the breast to the armpit. If the cancer spreads beyond the basement membrane of the lobule (the milk-producing glands) or ducts of the breast into the breast tissue, the woman risks the possibility of this cancer moving to the lymph nodes in the armpit and spreading to other areas of the body.

If the cancer has already spread to the lymph nodes, surgeons "upstage" the patient to at least Stage II. Invasive breast cancers are common; in 2010, about 126 cases of invasive breast cancer occurred for every 100,000 American women, according to the National Cancer Institute (NCI).[1,2]

Noninvasive Cancer

Surgeons debate whether to use sentinel node biopsy for patients with ductal carcinoma in situ, which has not spread beyond the walls of the milk ducts into the surrounding breast tissue. While this cancer is not life threatening (because it is not invasive), those with the disease may face a greater chance of developing invasive breast cancer later on if the DCIS is not properly treated.

Usually, if a patient has a small, low- or intermediate-grade in situ breast cancer, there's no reason to perform SNB. However, women with high-grade in situ breast cancer are another matter. High-grade ductal carcinoma in situ (DCIS) may be larger than seen on a mammogram and may also harbor small areas of invasive cancer. With larger high-grade DCIS, SNB is indicated. Noninvasive cancers are less common. In 2010, about 33 cases of in situ breast cancers occurred for every 100,000 American women, according to the NCI.[3]

Special Situations

When imaging studies suggest the presence of a large area of high-grade DCIS, the situation calls for focused attention. The larger the area of the high-grade DCIS, the more concerned doctors become about the possibility of an underlying invasive cancer that could spread to the lymph nodes.

"We could argue that if the patient chooses lumpectomy, and the surgeon discovers invasive cancer with the final pathology report, we can do sentinel node biopsy during a second surgery," Dr. Harness says. "If we do so, there's a little fall-off in accuracy of detection, because of the disruption of some of the lymphatic system in the breast. But when a patient chooses mastectomy, the surgeon can't go back and do a sentinel node biopsy after the procedure. Our bridges are burned. Therefore, a sentinel node biopsy is indicated with all mastectomies—for either invasive or noninvasive cancer."

Surgeons also currently debate whether there's a role for sentinel node biopsy in women selected to undergo prophylactic (preventive) mastectomy, a procedure often performed on healthy women who have a high risk of developing breast cancer in either breast. The current recommendation is not to do a sentinel node biopsy in the armpit on the uninvolved side if the imaging studies—mammogram, ultrasound, MRI—are negative.

The Pathology Report

On the day of the patient's breast cancer surgery, the work of the surgeon winds down after the surgery is completed, but the efforts of the pathologist continue. He or she performs an inventory of examinations of the tumor tissue and prepares a final report of the findings. In some cases, the breast, lymph nodes, and other tissue may also be sent out to another lab for further examination.

This final pathology report proves critical in the staging of breast cancers after surgery, and helps influence later treatment options. This document provides information on whether a breast cancer is Stage 0, Stage I, Stage II, or at another stage, indicating the extent of cancer within the mammary gland and its spread to the lymph nodes. Ultimately, pathologists shoulder the critical responsibility of determining the stage of a patient's breast cancer.

A pathologist obtains considerable information by looking at breast tumor tissue under a microscope. He or she sends a report of findings to your surgeon, who can explain them to you. At the top of this report, the pathologist describes the examined tissue. The report includes the weight and dimensions of the excised tumor or tumors, and a description of how the tissue looked. Physicians call this a gross description, meaning it describes how the tumor looked to a trained observer without using a microscope.

The report also indicates whether cancer was found in just one area or in many areas of the breast, and it will say whether cancer cells traveled to the skin or nipple. It also states whether the tumor was lodged on the chest wall, and whether microcalcifications (calcium deposits) were found.

Your Cancer Fingerprint

The pathology report helps establish the "fingerprint" of your breast cancer. Over time, this fingerprint helps your treatment team answer several questions:

- How aggressively do your breast cancer cells behave?

- Have any cancer cells migrated from the original tumor and traveled elsewhere, such as under the arm into the lymph nodes?

- Does the cancer contain biological features that indicate whether or not it will respond to certain cancer treatments?

Once the pathologist slips tumor tissue under a microscope, the device magnifies it hundreds of times and shows details of tissue previously stained to enhance the appearance of certain details.

What the pathologist finds may vary a bit from the findings of the core biopsy, which was performed before your breast cancer surgery and took only a small amount of tissue from your breast. After your surgery, he or she examines a much greater amount of tissue, which yields much more information.

For example, different types of cancer can and do commonly reside in the breast. Taking tissue from the greater expanse of excised tumor is more likely to capture cells of multiple malignant types. For that reason, most of the time, the pathologist can determine any type of breast cancer removed from your breast during surgery.

Widespread vs. Focal

Chances are the pathologist will submit a report that describes your cancer as ductal carcinoma or lobular carcinoma, which tells you whether the cells most likely arose in the duct or the lobule. Some cancers contain a mix of cells from both ducts and lobules.

Moving on, the report may then list whether the cancer is invasive. If not, the pathologist labels it as ductal carcinoma in situ; intraductal carcinoma; lobular carcinoma in situ; or non-invasive carcinoma.

Invasive or infiltrating cancers are those that have escaped the duct or lobule. Reports on these cancers specify invasive ductal (or lobular) carcinoma or infiltrating ductal (or lobular) carcinoma.

Cancers arising in the ducts and lobules are also referred to as *adenocarcinomas*, a broad term describing a bigger category of malignancies. Other names for cancers may also appear on the pathologist's report. For the most part they're variations on invasive ductal cancer, labeled by the pathologist according to how the cells look under the microscope.

The Tumor in Your Breast: How Aggressive Is It?

After identifying the type of cancer you have, the pathologist looks at its cells very carefully. He or she is inspecting their appearance. Various cancer cells show different degrees of differentiation. The cells are not the same, and they don't act the same way. Just like thugs in a bad neighborhood, cancer cells exhibit different levels of aggressiveness. High-grade tumors, for example, exhibit more aggressive cells.

Differentiation

Wild-looking cells, also called poorly differentiated cells, usually act more aggressively than those with a more normal appearance, which are referred to as well differentiated. Cells that fall in between these extremes are defined as moderately differentiated.

Tubules

Breast cancers form tubules in ductal cancers but not lobular cancers, and the pathologist examines the cells to gain information about the degree of tubular formation. Well-shaped tubules may suggest a better prognosis.

Mitosis

The pathologist also examines the slides to learn how many of the tumor's cells are dividing and the rate at which they are doing so, a process known as *mitotic rate* or activity. Observing highly aggressive cells often reveals that many cells are dividing at the same time, which reflects more rapid growth of these cells. Fewer cells are dividing in less aggressive tumors.

Nuclear Grade

Closely related to tumor growth and differentiation is a tumor's nuclear grade. Inside the cell is a nucleus containing DNA, and the grade reflects just how abnormal the DNA is. Your DNA is graded on a scale from 1 to 3 or 1 to 4, and the higher the grade, the more serious the situation.

Vessels

The pathologist looks for other signs of aggression in the thug inside your body. He or she looks to see if cancer cells are inside blood or lymphatic vessels. If the specialist finds cancer cells there, there will be vascular invasion, lymphatic invasion, or lymphovascular invasion, which implies that the cancer could be more dangerous than others.

A very thorough physician, the pathologist sometimes tracks the number of blood or lymph vessels associated with the tumor. A large number of blood vessels may signal rapid doubling of tumor cells. This is because tumors secrete substances that cause blood vessels to grow, a process called *angiogenesis* or *lymphangeogenesis* (growth of new lymphatics). A large concentration of blood vessels may indicate that the tumor is growing more rapidly and thus is especially aggressive.

Examining all these factors vastly expands the available information about the cancer. All the data helps define the nature of the cells in your tumor, but no one examination predicts the behavior of any cell all the time. In an attempt to be accurate, the results of the pathologist's observations are combined into a score.

Scoring

A commonly used scoring system is the Nottingham histologic score, otherwise known as the modified Scarff-Bloom-Richardson score. When you find a Nottingham or Scarff-Bloom-Richardson score on your report, you know your pathologist used a certain method for measuring how your tumor looked.

Staging

The pathologist's report also lists staging information. Stage I tumors measure up to 2 centimeters, but cancer cells have not yet invaded the lymph nodes. Stage II tumors may be lymph node positive or lymph node negative, but they measure between 2 and 5 centimeters.

Stage III tumors are commonly divided into subcategories A, B, and C. For IIIA, the cancer is typically 5 centimeters or greater and has spread to lymph nodes, and there are one to three lymph nodes that contain cancer. You can also be stage IIIA with any size tumor and with four to nine lymph nodes that contain cancer. For IIIB, the cancer can be of any size, with a tumor growing in the chest wall and/or the skin in the breast.

There may be no lymph nodes that contain cancer, or multiple lymph nodes may be cancerous. For IIIC, cancer may not be visible in the breast, but if it is, it may be of any size. The tumor may have spread to the chest wall and/or the skin in the breast. Such cancer may have spread to lymph nodes located above or below the collarbone, and ten or more nodes may contain cancer.

Margins

Another important aspect of the pathologist's report involves whether the margins around the tumor were free of cancer. This information helps predict how much cancer may still exist in the breast. A positive margin usually means more tissue needs to be removed.

Lymph Nodes

The pathologist's summary report also includes how many lymph nodes removed or sampled showed cancer. The number of lymph nodes removed is also shown.

Look Behind

Subtle but important differences in cancer cells aren't always easily seen on slides viewed under the microscope. Because of the challenges, pathologists sometimes ask other pathologists to provide a second opinion of an analysis. This is an easy exercise in a hospital with multiple pathologists, but not so simple in a rural hospital with a small staff.

Patients can sometimes arrange to have pathologists at a larger hospital nearby reexamine slides from their breast tumor, and slides can be sent from your hospital to the larger hospital for this purpose. In some cases, your slides can be digitally scanned and sent to the nearby pathology department over the Internet. This is true globally.

Other Examinations

The pathologist also begins working up a molecular profile of your cancer. He or she reports on whether the tumor has markers that are positive or negative for estrogen, progesterone, or HER-2-neu. Each of these indicators has implications for the adjuvant therapy you receive. The pathologist may also report on the presence of a Ki-67 marker that indicates how rapidly cells are dividing.

Genomic Analysis

In some cases, the pathologist sends tumor tissues off for a genomic analysis (a profile of some of the genes in the cancer itself). Such tests may be used to help determine chemotherapy and radiation therapy options. In some cases patients can forgo chemotherapy or radiation based on this analysis. Such tests currently include Oncotype DX, MammaPrint, and MammaStrat, but others are being developed.

Radiation Oncologist

Another cancer specialist, the radiation oncologist, may also watch over you while you're in surgery. This specialist represents another guide accompanying you on your path. This doctor specializes in delivering radiation therapy. Research shows that receiving focused radiation to the tumor bed may increase the effectiveness of whole-breast radiation treatment (described in Chapter 8). This is called the "boost." The boost can be done at the time of surgery or at the end of a course of whole-breast radiation therapy. With conventional approaches, women receive whole breast radiation sometime after surgery, which would include the boost if it was not done at the time of surgery. Treatment lasts four to six weeks. Radiation is thought to kill off tiny tumors so small that no medical image and no examination of tumor tissue can identify them.

At an increasing number of U.S. centers, women are benefiting from a treatment innovation known as *intraoperative radiation therapy* (IORT). They receive a single fraction (dose) of radiation therapy at the time of surgery. But clinical scientists are still learning about this therapy, and its use has not become standard practice. As a result, most centers in the United States providing single-fraction IORT do so under research protocols.

This treatment, known as *intraoperative radiation therapy* (IORT), is planned by radiation oncologists in collaboration with breast surgeons. Where IORT is used, these specialists provide important treatment in operating rooms. Equipped with a portable unit, they enter the operating room with a physicist who calculates the optimal method of administering a radiation treatment to the patient while the skin on her breast is open and the tumor bed can be directly radiated.[4,5,6] On the day of your surgery, you'll be asleep under anesthesia when this oncologist shows up.

European surgeons and radiation oncologists use IORT more frequently than doctors in America. Research conducted in Salzburg, Austria suggests that combining a radiation boost on the day of surgery with whole breast radiation after surgery reduces the rate of breast cancer recurrence. Clinicians at University Hospital Salzburg of Paracelsus Private Medical School studied 387 women with Stage I or II breast cancer who opted for surgery that saved their breasts. One hundred ninety of the women were given a radiation boost (IORT, 9 Gy)[7] to the area of their tumor during surgery. Radiation oncologists later gave them whole breast radiation (51–56 Gy). Another 188 women, very much like the other subjects in age, menopausal status, tumor grade and size, and status of lymph nodes, completed surgery and radiation to the whole breast (51–56 Gy), and then received a radiation boost (12 Gy). Over five years, women given a radiation boost at the time of surgery with whole breast radiation after surgery developed very few new cancers in the same breast. Recurrence was at zero percent. Cancer recurred in 4.3 percent of the women who received the alternate protocol used in the study.[8]

The use of IORT in the treatment of breast cancer is not appropriate for all cases. Patient selection for the use of this technology is very important in achieving good outcomes. As the results of clinical trials and large institutional series become more available, it will become clearer which patients can safely undergo single-fraction IORT as an appropriate method for performing partial breast irradiation therapy.

Endnotes

1. Breast cancer incidence rates were age-adjusted to the "2000 US Std Population," the NCI reported.

2. Howlader N, Noone AM, Krapcho M, Garshell J, Neyman N, Altekruse SF, Kosary CL, Yu M, Ruhl J, Tatalovich Z, Cho H, Mariotto A, Lewis DR, Chen HS, Feuer EJ, Cronin KA (eds). SEER Cancer Statistics Review, 1975-2010, National Cancer Institute. Bethesda. Available at seer.cancer.gov/csr/1975_2010/, based on Nov 2012 SEER data submission, posted to the SEER web site, 2013.

3. Ibid.

4. Vaidya, JS. Targeted intraoperative radiotherapy versus whole breast radiotherapy for breast cancer (TARGIT A Trial): an international, prospective, randomized, non-inferiority phase 3 trial. Lancet 2010; 376 (July): 91-102.

5. Khan, AJ. Ultrashort Courses of Adjuvant Breast Radiotherapy. Wave of the Future or Fool's Errand? Cancer 2011 (August 27).

6. Vaidya, JS. Long-term results of targeted intraoperative radiotherapy (TARGIT) boost during breast-conserving surgery. *Int J Radiation Oncology Biol Phy* 2011; 81:1091-1097.

7. Radiation oncologists measure units known as Grays (Gy). A Gray measures a unit of radiation dose of absorbed radiation, based on an international system of units used by scientists across the globe.

8. Retsamer R, et al. The Salzburg concept of intraoperative radiotherapy for breast cancer: results and considerations. *Int J Cancer* 2006; 118(11):2882-2887.

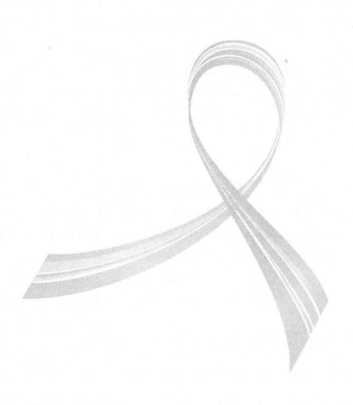

Chapter 5

Listening: Emotionally Preparing for Surgery

When cancer arises in the body, women sometimes recognize that it's there. The knowing is at a subconscious level, but the body does begin to speak, and it behooves women to listen to it. Some women have vivid dreams full of warning symbols. One woman with undiagnosed breast cancer dreamed of being in a biplane flown by a daring pilot who conducted maneuvers fraught with danger. She then painted a picture of a disappearing tree. This woman was Phyllis Gapen, the coauthor of this book.

As the pathologist and other doctors interpret tests, they also begin listening to a woman's body. What they "hear" from these tests guides treatment choices and ultimately influences what the breast becomes.

As the surgeon works, he or she creates solutions that transform lives. Outcomes echo the wisdom imparted in an ancient Chinese fable:

A stone carver, Hung Liu, created animal sculptures from colored stone. "How do you know what to carve?" an observer asked him.

"I always approach the stone," the carver replied. "The stone tells me what nature left to reveal." He went on with his work of carving animals.

When one of the Ming emperors wanted a green and white jade stone carved into a fierce dragon and several dogs, the carver was summoned and asked to shape the fearsome beasts.

When the carver shifted his awareness and attuned himself to the patterns of the universe remaining in the jade, a problem immediately arose. Nature had left in the stone a pattern of a carp, a fish that darts swiftly through water.

With reluctance, knowing it could lead to his downfall, the carver told the emperor that the exquisite jade stone wanted to become a school of carp. When the emperor realized the artist wanted to carve something other than a fierce dragon, he was livid. His advisors suggested punishment for the artist, but slowly the emperor began to realize the carver had merely recognized the creatures yearning to emerge from the stone. He asked the carver to follow his instinct. Eventually the emperor came to prize the jade carving of the carp, and he sent the carver home to continue carving what nature had left in the stone.[1]

So it is with sculpting a human breast invaded by cancer. The surgery that is chosen isn't what a woman would ever have wanted to undergo, but carefully selected and creatively executed procedures address her specific cancer and remove it from her body. With modern diagnostic and treatment tools and reconstructive breast surgery, her body can be beautiful and healthy, even though her breast is changed. She can live and embrace life with greater awareness and with mastery.

A woman's breast or breasts will never look or feel the same after breast surgery. But with a skillful surgeon performing an artful, carefully selected procedure, she can obtain a better outcome.

The selection of this doctor and the formal or informal medical teams that he or she practices with marks a critical juncture on a woman's cancer journey. For many reasons, the outcomes of breast surgeries are highly variable. Some surgeons are uncomfortable with or untrained in special techniques that improve cosmetic outcomes, and are unable to provide them. Still others feel most comfortable performing only a small range of techniques because they are familiar with and adept at those techniques.

When surgeons reconstruct breasts, they use surgical techniques developed for breast cancer patients. These techniques are called *oncoplastic*—from *onco*, meaning cancer, and *plastic*, referring to plastic surgery—and they require considerable experience and training. Oncoplastic techniques first remove cancer. But the strategies go far beyond the boundaries of cosmetic surgery for the breast—they *create* a new, aesthetically pleasing breast shape.

To achieve a satisfactory outcome, a woman should strive to align her vision with the skills and preferences of a surgeon attuned to the signals revealed as her cancer is probed by her treatment team.

Choices

Many women encounter similar cancer scenarios. Large numbers face cancer that is spreading outside the milk ducts and must be stopped. In 2011, nearly 80 percent of all American women diagnosed with breast cancer dealt with an invasive ductal carcinoma, according to the National Cancer Institute's SEER database. Their cancer presented in different ways.

The nature of a woman's cancer determines the type of cancer surgery she receives and the reconstructive surgery choices available to her. Its characteristics shape the possibilities for what the breast can become. Like Hung Liu, the surgeon artfully considers how to proceed given the medium he or she has to work with and the options for shaping it.

When women undergo lumpectomy, the surgeon removes the tumor and some of the normal tissue that surrounds it. This strategy helps preserve the breast.

Cosmetic results depend on both tumor size and breast size. Taking a large tumor out of a sizable breast may leave a normal-appearing breast, but eliminating a large tumor from a small breast can produce noticeable and unacceptable changes in the size and shape of the breast. Oncoplasty may be able to compensate for these changes.

"During lumpectomy surgery in my practice, we move healthy tissue inside the breast so that any indention that remains from the removal of breast cancer fills up," Dr. Harness explains. "Afterward, the breast maintains its normal shape, or displays a better one."

Large-breasted women undergoing lumpectomy often seek to regain symmetry afterward, and are rebalanced.

With a mastectomy, the breast is removed entirely, taking the whole tumor with it. But this isn't your grandmother's mastectomy, an operation so extensive that women feared it greatly. Skillful surgeons now attempt to preserve as much skin and muscle as possible, and in some cases can provide skin-sparing or nipple-sparing mastectomies.

"During mastectomy surgery, we reconstruct the breast with tissue from other parts of the body or use a tissue expander, which is later replaced with an implant," Dr. Harness says. "This helps the woman regain her beauty. Reconstruction often begins immediately at the time of the first breast surgery; surgeons perform it in two stages. The woman returns later for more procedures that restore her. These may include procedures that achieve symmetry for both breasts."

Some women undergoing mastectomy decline reconstructive surgery. In such cases, the woman's skin is pulled tight under the arm and the chest area is made flat. A breast prosthesis then fits artfully over the chest wall to give the appearance of a breast under the patient's clothing.

The chart below shows some of the surgical options available to women with ductal carcinoma in situ and other diagnoses. Keep in mind that not all women with the same diagnosis receive the same treatment. The stage of their cancer, its molecular fingerprint, and its genomic structure influence treatment options, including the type of reconstructive surgery that will be performed. This chart does NOT list all possible options or details.

Like explorers, the medical team sometimes uses information obtained from the pathologist's report that follows breast surgery to redraw the map used for the next stages of a woman's cancer journey. With the cancerous tumor out of the body, new information may dictate a better path that achieves the best outcome.

General Considerations and Treatment Scenarios

Ductal Carcinoma In Situ (DCIS)	Surgery	Radiation	Reconstruction
Typically found with mammography. Core biopsy obtained. ER, PR status determined. If ER or PR positive, treat with anti-estrogen therapy for five years after the completion of initial surgery and radiation therapy.	If localized, use lumpectomy to remove affected area, obtaining clear margins around the tumor.	Often follow up with radiation therapy in most cases.	Oncoplastic techniques to achieve good cosmetic result.
Mastectomy for DCIS	**Surgery**	**Radiation**	**Reconstruction**
	Generally done with extensive DCIS or patient choice.	No radiation therapy.	Reconstruction with implants or autologous tissue (a flap of your own tissue from the abdominal wall or back).

Lobular Carcinoma In Situ (LCIS)	Surgery	Radiation	Reconstruction
LCIS is usually not considered a cancer, but is a marker lesion for the increased risk of subsequent cancer. Close monitoring, chance of developing invasive cancer is 1 percent per year in either breast. Incidental finding when breast surgery performed for another reason. Depending on other factors, taking tamoxifen or raloxifene (postmenopausal) for five years can be used as a strategy to prevent or delay future development of cancer.	Close observation.	Radiation therapy, chemotherapy not needed.	

Invasive Ductal Carcinoma	Surgery	Radiation	Reconstruction
	If localized, perform lumpectomy. Mastectomy may be needed for larger tumors or multicentric disease involving other parts of the breast or patient choice.	Radiation therapy if lumpectomy performed. Appropriate chemotherapy and anti-hormonal therapy.	Reconstruction with implants or autologous tissue after mastectomy.

Invasive Lobular Carcinoma	Surgery	Radiation	Reconstruction
Typically, all tumors are ER positive, HER-2-neu negative.	If localized, perform lumpectomy. Mastectomy may be needed for larger tumors or patient choice.	Radiation therapy, chemotherapy as indicated. Take appropriate anti-hormonal therapy.	Oncoplastic techniques. Reconstruction, implant or autologous tissue.

Reconstructive Techniques

Surgeons use a number of reconstructive techniques to shape the remaining breast or a new one. An overview of some of these techniques is included here.

Implants

During breast cancer surgery, a surgeon places a tissue expander underneath or on top of the pectoralis muscle of the chest wall. This expander is then inflated with salt water (saline solution) in a series of visits to the plastic surgeon. Later, a silicone or saline implant may replace the inflated saline tissue expander.

Flaps

Breast reconstruction with flap surgery involves taking a section of tissue from one area of your body and relocating it to your chest area to form a new breast. In a latissimus dorsi flap procedure, a surgeon removes a muscle and some skin from the upper back and uses it to reconstruct the breast. Women with large breasts often also get a permanent silicone implant under the flap that balances the size and shape of both breasts.

With a TRAM (Transverse Rectus Abdominis Myocutaneous) flap procedure, a surgeon places a thick section of abdominal skin, fat, and muscle to be used at the mastectomy site. This procedure may transplant part of the transverse rectus abdominus muscle found in the abdominal wall. Tissue transplants occur using one of two approaches:

A pedicle TRAM flap moves tissue from the belly to the

chest in a process that requires tunneling it under the skin while its blood vessels remain attached.

A free TRAM flap involves trimming the skin, fat, and muscle from the abdomen, along with its blood vessels. Tissue is moved and blood vessels reattached to new ones at the mastectomy site.

With a DIEP flap procedure, a surgeon removes abdominal skin, fat, and blood vessels, but preserves muscle from the upper abdominal wall. The surgeon identifies perforator vessels that split off from an artery and vein deep in the body and travel through the muscle before arriving in the fat and the skin. The plastic surgeon separates out these vessels and trims them out of the tissue by going through the muscle, instead of excising the muscle containing these small vessels. No muscle is removed. This work is so exacting that a microscope must be used to reconnect the blood supply to the deep inferior epigastric perforator (DIEP) flap used to shape the new breast. Women who undergo this procedure sometimes report that they eventually regain some sensation in the breast. They also enjoy a shorter recovery time and endure less pain.

Symmetry

A mastopexy is a special procedure that lifts the breast on the opposite side to create symmetry in the breasts following mastectomy. It is often performed months after the first stage of reconstructive surgery. On the mastectomy side, it may also be used to lift sagging skin.

For women with large breasts, surgeons sometimes reduce the size of both the affected breast and the opposite, unaffected breast in order to achieve an attractive symmetry.

The patient and her surgeon decide which of these techniques to use, and whether to utilize implants. The majority of women who opt for reconstruction now get saline or silicone implants, rather than transplants of their own tissue.

Delaying or Proceeding With Reconstruction

The woman and her surgeon also confer on whether to use reconstructive techniques immediately after breast surgery or at a later time.

The decision to delay or proceed immediately depends on many factors, such as the stage of your cancer, your general medical status, your lifestyle and preferences, and other therapies you require to treat your cancer (such as radiation therapy). Most breast surgeons advocate for the use of first-stage reconstruction with a tissue expander at the time of mastectomy.

When skin can be spared during a mastectomy, surgeons often use it as a pocket for a flap or an expander that creates an attractive new shape. Obtaining good surgical results is simpler if a woman doesn't need radiation therapy.

For women who do need it, postsurgical radiation therapy can introduce complex issues for surgeons doing reconstruction, but specialists minimize the challenges. Right after a skin-sparing mastectomy, surgeons may place a tissue expander inside the remaining envelope of breast skin and inflate it with saline to stretch the skin and muscle before the woman begins radiation therapy. This prepares the breast mound for the second stage of reconstruction. Several months after radiation therapy ends, the woman may receive a permanent saline or silicone implant, depending on her circumstances and preferences.

In different medical centers, a variety of techniques are used for expanding first-stage implants for women who need radiation therapy. How much expansion is done and how late it is done in the treatment process depends on the preferences of the treatment team. If expansion begins after the conclusion of radiation therapy, it needs to be started promptly, before fibrosis (extra scarring tissue) of the irradiated skin begins to develop.

Women who must undergo radiation treatment may be advised to use their own tissue (with or without an implant) when they opt for delayed reconstruction. If they choose to use their own tissue (autologous tissue) to help build the breast mound, standard treatment calls for placing flaps of tissue in the mound after radiation treatment ends, to avoid damaging such important tissue.

Advantages and Disadvantage of Immediate and Delayed Reconstruction

Women who have the option to undergo immediate or delayed reconstruction may find that evaluating the advantages and disadvantages of both surgeries helps them to arrive at a decision.

Advantages/Immediate Reconstruction	Disadvantages/ Immediate Reconstruction
• Patient never experiences being without a breast shape. • Improved cosmetic results. • Fewer likely surgeries, reduced costs. • Other treatments, such as chemotherapy, are not delayed.	• Woman may spend more time in the hospital than when mastectomy alone is performed. • Woman spends longer time recovering than if she only undergoes mastectomy. • Woman may emerge from mastectomy surgery with more scars and possibly additional complications.
Advantages/Delayed Reconstruction	**Disadvantages/Delayed Reconstruction**
• Patient gains more time to consider reconstruction options. • If a woman opted for radiation therapy, she may need to undergo delayed reconstruction with autologous tissue. • If a woman needs chemotherapy, she can proceed with needed treatment and delay reconstruction. • Any issues that arise with skin flaps, such as necrosis, are resolved, as tissue has healed.	• Patient lives with a scar on her chest wall. • Additional surgery and recovery time required.

Talking to Doctors, Getting Support

Before undergoing surgery, ask your surgeon for photographs of the breasts of women who have completed breast surgery and reconstruction in his or her practice.

If you opt for a mastectomy, and you need radiation therapy and want reconstruction, meet with a plastic surgeon and a radiation oncologist prior to undergoing the mastectomy. Going over reconstruction options with these physicians ensures that you understand how your choice for breast surgery affects the reconstructive procedures available to you.

Find out whether the surgeon and plastic surgeon you turn to have privileges to practice in the hospital where you are being treated. This is especially important if you want immediate reconstruction.

If you haven't selected a plastic surgeon, you can locate one in your area by contacting the American Society of Plastic Surgeons. The group's phone number is 800-514-5058, and its website is plasticsurgery.org.

While you decide which is the best surgical course, be gentle with yourself. You have a lot to consider. To help you make decisions, you may want to try guided imagery, a form of daydreaming, to envision your responses to the challenges and outcomes of possible surgical solutions. Such imaging promotes healing by focusing the mind on how it looks, feels, and sounds to have a desired experience. Such reveries give a cancer patient a sense of being in control when things seem out of control.

Embrace the fact that life has made you a manager; you're making critical choices about your own life. How well you manage yourself, your medical treatment, and many aspects of your personal and work life will help shape your future.

You may find it helpful to talk to other patients who have undergone the operations you're considering. Among the things you'll discover from such talks: Modern reconstruction can produce beautiful results, but multiple operations may be required, and women will experience some postoperative pain while they heal from special operations. Recovering from procedures that use flaps to form newly shaped breasts can require six weeks of healing. Over time, however, the scars from your surgery will fade.

The Livestrong Foundation provides one-on-one telephone counseling to cancer patients and links them to support groups. You can call them at 855-220-777 or go to livestrong.org/we-can-help. The foundation also partners with Imerman Angels (imermanangels.org) to offer these support services. You can contact Imerman Angels at 877-274-5529.

The National Cancer Institute's Cancer Information Service (800-4-CANCER or 800-422-6237; cancer.gov/aboutnci) provides a list of support groups, as do local chapters of the American Cancer Society (cancer.org) and the Susan G. Komen for the Cure organization (komen.org). Another organization that offers information about support is CancerCare (cancercare.org).

SHARE, an organization based in New York City, helps connect breast cancer patients living in that region. SHARE's website is sharecancersupport.org, and its number is 866-892-2392.

Personnel at the hospital where you are being treated may also be able to help you find a support group in your area.

When you're ready, schedule a visit with your surgeon to talk about the choices you think are right for you, and work together to make a shared decision that satisfies both of you. The most appropriate surgical decisions depend on an assessment of relevant factors. If you're to undergo a mastectomy, the factors that influence reconstruction options include:

- The shape of your body

- Operations you've had in the past

- Your current health status

- Treatments you require

- Your own personal preferences

Like the jade carver, listen to your body, and dare to imagine what your breast wants to be. Embrace the fact that life has made you a manager; you're making critical choices about your own life. How well you manage yourself, your medical treatment, and many aspects of your personal and work life will help shape your future.

Endnotes

1. Gump AL. Jade, *Stone of Heaven*. New York: Doubleday & Co.; 1962: 85.

Chapter 6

Regaining Wholeness:
Emotional Reconstruction®

The personal history of every woman is intricately linked to her gender. When women learn they must undergo breast surgery for cancer, many of them discover how closely they identify their breasts with their sexuality. For them, the human breast symbolizes important aspects of femininity, including beauty.

A very obvious part of a woman's body that also remains private, the breast was linked to the sacred in Judeo Christian tradition. Believers thought the breast provided spiritual nourishment to Christian souls.[1] A shapely figure also held the possibility of healthy offspring.

The ancient Greeks linked the breast to vital aspects of the divine feminine nature. A multibreasted statue of Artemis of

Ephesus provided a symbol of generosity, productivity, and sensuality.[2, 3]

When the structure of an organ with the status of a cultural icon must change, a woman faces the challenge of finding a way to eventually feel contented with her body again. From the moment a woman gets a breast cancer diagnosis, she may struggle with her perception of her own desirability.

Even the simple act of planning for surgery pushes a woman to adjust to a new body image. Facing changes to the body often triggers anxiety.[4] Some women begin withdrawing emotionally and socially; others expand, facing their fear and embracing life and its possibilities.[5,6]

Pathways exist to make this adjustment easier for a woman with breast cancer. Women can help themselves by striving for a positive frame of mind as they process information about their cancer, make decisions about surgery, and prepare for it. For example, a woman's mind-set contributes to the outcome of her surgery. However, attaining a beneficial, relaxed, confident state of mind may take weeks.[7,8]

Exercise helps prepare the body for surgery and other treatments, as long as it matches the woman's energy level. Some women may find it helpful to talk gently and lovingly to their bodies while preparing to undergo breast surgery or reconstruction. Cancer coaches taught Phyllis Gapen, the coauthor of this book, to get ready for the event by standing naked in front of a mirror, thanking her body for its breasts, and offering gratitude for the beauty and service they had provided in this life. She was also advised to sing to her body and to use breathing exercises.

Addressing Cosmetic and Emotional Needs

Some surgeons have adapted the art of plastic surgery to address both the cosmetic concerns and the emotional needs of women with breast cancer. Today, a growing number of women can access surgeons skilled in oncoplastic surgery,

> *With each action undertaken in oncoplasty, the surgeon and his or her team seek to shape the whole woman.*

who embrace a philosophy that seeks to bring a woman back to a state of physical and emotional health after cancer. With each action undertaken in oncoplasty, the surgeon and his or her team seek to shape the whole woman.

With this approach, women often wake up after lumpectomy or mastectomy surgery and find that their breasts have an attractive shape.

"After oncoplastic surgery, the patient often displays a normal contour and sometimes the breast shape is even lovelier than before a lumpectomy," Dr. Harness says.

"With a mastectomy, oncoplastic techniques often help a woman quickly regain the figure she had before cancer surgery. Immediately after the first breast surgery, we often begin rebuilding the breast. We do this in stages."

When feasible, the surgeon saves a large amount of skin from the breast during the mastectomy. Doing so facilitates the use of a plastic tissue expander or tissue from other parts of the body. When an expander is used, a plastic surgeon gradually fills the flat bag with saline until it takes on the shape of a breast. The process takes weeks. Having access to a skin flap enables the surgical team to perform reconstruction that may produce a more natural-looking breast shape.[9,10,11]

Some mastectomies are done with techniques that spare the patient's breast skin, areola, and nipple. Thus, the woman leaves the operating suite with her own areola and nipple. The new breast usually displays a pleasing shape, although the woman loses sensation in the areola and nipple. Saving these structures achieves the best cosmetic result for the patient.

If the nipple cannot be saved during a mastectomy, a surgeon can reconstruct the structure several months after the initial surgery. A small flap of skin is used to shape the nipple and then tattooed with color to create the impression of the areola and the nipple on the tip of the breast.[12,13] These surgical practices help patients who may feel disfigured by breast cancer surgery.

Not every woman wants to take the first steps toward reconstruction at the time of her breast cancer surgery. Some wait for months or years. In fact, not all women want to undergo reconstruction.[14,15]

Some may simply opt to be fitted for a breast prosthesis made of silicone. Many of these soft, flexible "falsies" slip easily into a pocket in a special bra, resulting in the appearance of a breast as viewed underneath clothing. For women with large breasts, use of these breast forms may help reduce uneven strain on their backs after a mastectomy. For women with small breasts misshapen from breast surgery, breast forms may help restore their outward appearance while they decide among reconstruction options.[16,17,18]

If you're a woman who wants breast reconstruction, find out about your options, and seek out information about the possible benefits, risks, side effects, and results from the surgery. Reconstruction will not increase the risk of breast cancer recurrence or make it harder to find a cancer that returns. Your doctors will use appropriate tests to monitor you for recurrence.[19,20]

Factors that influence recurrence include:

- Initial stage of your cancer.

- The fingerprint of the cancer (ER, PR, and HER-2-neu status) and other biological characteristics.

- The modalities (surgery, chemotherapy, etc.) used to treat your breast cancer.

In most cases, undergoing reconstruction does not delay the start of any chemotherapy you may need.[21,22]

"If you need radiation therapy after a mastectomy, it can be done with a tissue expander in place," Dr. Harness says. "For example, if you want to complete reconstructive surgery using a skin flap, it is advisable to undergo radiation therapy and then wait at least four months after the end of this therapy to put a flap in place."[23,24]

Questions about Reconstruction

Patients should ask some probing questions before undergoing surgery that alters the breast:[25]

- Which reconstructive surgery do you recommend for me and why?

- Will my breasts be symmetrical after the reconstruction?

- Do you recommend any surgery for the healthy breast, in order to achieve symmetry?

- What scars will I have on my breast or breasts after the surgery?

- How many reconstructions like mine have you done?

- What kind of pain should I expect, and how long might it last?

- How will my reconstructed breast change over time?

- What complications or side effects are expected from this type of surgery?

- How many surgeries will be required?

- May I speak with a patient who has undergone the type of surgery you recommend?

Financing Reconstruction

Women who want reconstruction should check into the reconstructive procedures their health insurer finances and their share of the total costs of the surgeries.

Today, women frequently undergo reconstruction with expanders and implants and with latissimus dorsi flaps. Free TRAMs and DIEP flap reconstructions that use a woman's tissue to shape a new breast are often done at academic medical centers staffed with large surgical teams.[26,27] (Flap reconstructions were discussed in Chapter 5.)

The Women's Health and Cancer Rights Act of 1998—which was amended in 2001 to impose penalties for not following the law—requires group health insurance and individual insurers to provide coverage for reconstructive surgery after a mastectomy. Insurers must pay for:

- Reconstruction of a breast removed during mastectomy.

- Surgery on the other breast to produce symmetry.

- A prosthesis to replace the breast, and treatment of complications following the mastectomy.[28,29]

More and more women are opting for immediate breast reconstruction in the U.S. In recent years, the number of immediate breast reconstructions increased at an average rate of five percent a year. Implant use grew by an average of 11 percent a year, according to an analysis of data taken from the Nationwide Inpatient Sample database for 1998 to 2008.[30] Rates of reconstruction using a woman's own tissue did not change.

Survivorship Plan

Women who opt for reconstruction need a survivorship plan (see Chapter 11) to ensure that they receive needed follow-up care after cancer treatment. Women need mammograms on the healthy breast and possibly on the reconstructed one. For women with whose breasts have been reconstructed with implants, the Food and Drug Administration recommends obtaining an MRI once every three years. This exam reveals the status of the implant. Surgeons want to see their breast cancer patients annually to ensure the reconstruction remains in good order.

Patients should ask their surgeons what follow-up care they need if they opt for lumpectomy over mastectomy.[31,32,33]

A Satisfying Sexual Life

Reconstructing the body is an important step in helping a woman reclaim her wholeness. But communication helps in important transitions. Conversations with caregivers and with significant others help the woman begin to adjust to sexual realities that surface during treatment. Fatigue—and shyness about the new shape of her chest—may decrease a woman's desire for sex. Cuddling may replace lovemaking for a time, and eventually a lover may need to hold a woman differently due to side effects of treatment. Special strategies may be needed to make it possible to engage in intercourse with comfort and pleasure. Caregivers can help the patient learn what to do. Strategies include moisturizing and lubricating the vagina. Sexual toys may also be used.[34,35] Women may perform differently during sex following breast cancer surgery, but sexual pleasure remains possible.

A woman needs to feel good about herself to engage in a fulfilling sexual life. Finding the inner strength to go on after cancer treatment—and finding the discipline to take the steps necessary to thrive—fuels self-confidence and contributes to a full life including one with satisfying sex.[36,37]

Endnotes

1. Jones, DP. Cultural Views of the Female Breast. ABNF Jour 2004; Jan/Feb: 15-21.

2. Ibid.

3. Thibeault C, Sabo BM. Art, archetypes and alchemy: images of self-following treatment for breast cancer. Eur J Oncol Nurs 2012; April 16(2): 153-157.

4. Wells RW. Body image and surgical operations. AORN Jour 1975; April 21 (5):812-815

5. Arman M, et al. Living with breast cancer: a challenge to expansive and creative forces. Eur Jrnl Can Care 2002; 11:290-296.

6. Thibeault C, Sabo BM. "I'm still who I was" creating meaning through engagement in art: the experience of two breast cancer survivors. Eur J Oncol Nurs 2012; July 16(3):203-211.

7. Shockney, L. Stealing Second Base: A Breast Cancer Survivor's Experience and Breast Cancer Expert's Story. Sudbury, MA: Jones & Bartlett Learning, 2007.

8. Siegel B. *Love, Medicine, and Miracles.* New York City: Harper Collins, 1998.

9. Breast Reconstruction. Is it right for you? Boston: Health Dialog. Foundation for Informed Medical Decision Making, 2009.

10. Reshaping You: Breast Reconstruction for Breast Cancer Patients. Patient Education Office, M.D. Anderson Cancer Center; May 1, 2010. Patient education guides.

11. Weiss, EH, ed. Frankly Speaking About Cancer: Breast Reconstruction. Washington, DC: Cancer Support Community, 2011.

12. Reshaping You: Breast Reconstruction for Breast Cancer Patients. Patient Education Office, M.D. Anderson Cancer Center; May 1, 2010. Patient education guides.

13. Weiss, EH, ed. Frankly Speaking About Cancer: Breast Reconstruction. Washington, DC: Cancer Support Community, 2011.

14. Reshaping You: Breast Reconstruction for Breast Cancer Patients. Patient Education Office, M.D. Anderson Cancer Center; May 1, 2010. Patient education guides.

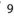

15. Weiss, EH, ed. Frankly Speaking About Cancer: Breast Reconstruction. Washington, DC: Cancer Support Community, 2011.

16. Shockney, L. Stealing Second Base: A Breast Cancer Survivor's Experience and Breast Cancer Expert's Story. Sudbury, MA: Jones & Bartlett Learning, 2007.

17. Reshaping You: Breast Reconstruction for Breast Cancer Patients. Patient Education Office, M.D. Anderson Cancer Center; May 1, 2010. Patient education guides.

18. Weiss, EH, ed. Frankly Speaking About Cancer: Breast Reconstruction. Washington, DC: Cancer Support Community, 2011.

19. Reshaping You: Breast Reconstruction for Breast Cancer Patients. Patient Education Office, M.D. Anderson Cancer Center; May 1, 2010. Patient education guides.

20. Weiss, EH, ed. Frankly Speaking About Cancer: Breast Reconstruction. Washington, DC: Cancer Support Community, 2011.

21. Reshaping You: Breast Reconstruction for Breast Cancer Patients. Patient Education Office, M.D. Anderson Cancer Center; May 1, 2010. Patient education guides.

22. Weiss, EH, ed. Frankly Speaking About Cancer: Breast Reconstruction. Washington, DC: Cancer Support Community, 2011.

23. Reshaping You: Breast Reconstruction for Breast Cancer Patients. Patient Education Office, M.D. Anderson Cancer Center; May 1, 2010. Patient education guides.

24. Weiss, EH, ed. Frankly Speaking About Cancer: Breast Reconstruction. Washington, DC: Cancer Support Community, 2011.

25. Reshaping You: Breast Reconstruction for Breast Cancer Patients. Patient Education Office, M.D. Anderson Cancer Center; May 1, 2010. Patient education guides.

26. Ibid.

27. Weiss, EH, ed. Frankly Speaking About Cancer: Breast Reconstruction. Washington, DC: Cancer Support Community, 2011.

28. Reshaping You Breast Reconstruction for Breast Cancer Patients. Patient Education Office, M.D. Anderson Cancer Center; May 1, 2010. Patient education guides.

29. Weiss, EH, ed. Frankly Speaking About Cancer: Breast Reconstruction. Washington, DC: Cancer Support Community, 2011

30. Albornoz, CR, et al. A Paradigm Shift in U.S. Breast Reconstruction: Increasing Implant Rates. Plast Reconstr Surg 2013; Jan 131(1):15–23.

31. Breast Reconstruction. Is it right for you? Boston: Health Dialog. Foundation for Informed Medical Decision Making, 2009.

32. Reshaping You: Breast Reconstruction for Breast Cancer Patients. Patient Education Office, M.D. Anderson Cancer Center; May 1, 2010. Patient education guides.

33. Weiss, EH, ed. Frankly Speaking About Cancer: Breast Reconstruction. Washington, DC: Cancer Support Community, 2011.

34. Shockney, L. Stealing Second Base: A Breast Cancer Survivor's Experience and Breast Cancer Expert's Story. Sudbury, MA: Jones & Bartlett Learning, 2007.

35. Krychman, ML, Kellogg Spade, S, Finestone, S. About Breast Cancer Sensuality, Sexuality and Intimacy. Sudbury, MA: Jones & Bartlett Learning, 2011.

36. Ibid.

37. Shockney, L. Stealing Second Base: A Breast Cancer Survivor's Experience and Breast Cancer Expert's Story. Sudbury, MA: Jones & Bartlett Learning, 2007.

Chapter 7

Systemic Therapy: Chemotherapy, Targeted Therapy, and Anti-Hormonal Therapy

From the outside, the female breast changes visibly over a lifetime. It buds in adolescence, produces milk during and after pregnancy, adjusts its shape after breastfeeding ends, and often loses definition as age advances.

On the inside, unseen changes happen constantly in its shifting environment. Profound alterations occur in mutated breast cells and in genes meant to suppress cancer. Scientists know that thousands of molecular and genetic changes in cells lead to breast cancer. New insights tell us that cancer of the breast is more than a cellular disease; it represents a molecular and genetic process.[1,2]

In the future, cancers may be more usefully classified according to their genetic mutations than by where they originate—i.e., the breast or the lungs. This idea comes out of new research, but must be proven.[3]

Mutations occur over a tumor's lifetime, but they likely emerge in just a fraction of tumor cells. Some of the first cancerous breast cells may be long-lived, dormant cells that are capable of multiplying rapidly when certain genetic changes occur. They may begin multiplying from a single or small number of cancer stem cells. The most potent of them may survive treatment with chemotherapy and radiation and go dormant for years afterward.[4]

From these cells may come less potent "generations" of cells, so that families of mutated cells make up the majority of cancerous tumor cells in the breast. The presence of such generations leads physicians to treat the body for cancer by addressing the circulation of cancer cells throughout the body. This is what is known as systemic therapy for invasive cancer.[5]

Signs of these flawed generations can be tracked. Errors occur in the living software of the human body. Thousands of genes supply coded information that creates thousands of proteins (molecules) that characterize a breast cell's structure and behavior. Only a small fraction of these codes transmit mutations with bad information that transforms normal cells into cancerous ones.[6,7]

When the body fails to correct its bad instructions or "software," these errors can trigger an over or under manufacture of important proteins that perform surveillance functions. Some of these proteins regulate a cell's growth and its behavior, and when they don't do so properly, the cell can become malignant or cancerous. Genes designed to stop flawed cells may fail.

Moreover, factors in the environment of the breast influence tumor development. The presence of estrogen in the breast is one of these factors.[8,9]

The most effective current therapies against potent cancer cells work by finding the mutated cancer cells that exert the greatest control over tumor development. These therapies may also alter the environment that supports these powerful cells. Successful treatment requires applying the right kind of treatment for the specific tumor.[10]

Treatments impact the whole body. "We've known for over thirty years that with invasive breast cancer, we have to treat the whole body, primarily because of cells elsewhere in the body that have been shed by the tumor and begun to circulate," Dr. Harness says.

New research has underscored the importance of this approach. A study at M.D. Anderson Cancer Center in Houston showed that breast cancer cells circulate in the body even in some women whose cancer cells have not spread to other organs. "Women with circulating cancer cells in the bloodstream face a higher risk of recurrence," Dr. Harness explains.[11,12]

"Those women in the study who had one or more detected circulating tumor cells had four times greater risk of their cancer coming back—and of course with recurrence the potential of dying."[13,14]

Finding the best treatment for these and other women isn't easy, Dr. Harness says. "But studies like this one at M.D. Anderson, published by Dr. Anthony Lucci and his team in

June 2012, will eventually allow us to begin to stratify patients to specific treatments that help them."

Altered cells that escape the protective measures of the human immune system pose challenges to developing medications that prevent breast cancer cells from dividing and invading. Researchers look for ways to hit cancer cells without damaging normal cells.

They also seek measures to control the environment in the breast. One way of doing this may be to lower inflammation in the body to inhibit processes that promote cancer. Exercise can push down levels of C-reactive protein, which is intimately linked to inflammation; consuming a heart-healthy diet can also improve the environment in the breast. Doctors also shift the environmental conditions in the body by using medications to block estrogen inside the breast.

Chemotherapy

Cancer spreads microscopically. Early on, it cannot be seen. When cancer cells escape the ducts and lobules, doctors suspect there are micrometastases, and in many cases, eliminating them becomes very important. To prevent these micrometastases from forming tumors in locations outside the breast, oncologists advise women with invasive cancer to undergo chemotherapy and/or anti-hormonal therapy. These treatments send drugs through the bloodstream to extend their reach to almost everywhere in the body.

Chemotherapy can be given before surgery (neoadjuvant therapy) to reduce the size of the tumor and determine whether the chemotherapy regimen works, or it can be administered after surgery (adjuvant therapy).

The selection of drugs used to treat you depends on the grade, hormone receptor status, size, and growth rate of your tumor, as well as your age, health, and menopausal status, and whether your lymph nodes contain cancer. Many drugs exist to treat breast cancer. Treatment plans typically call for using combinations of chemotherapy drugs. Your drugs have two names: the generic (or chemical) term for the drug and the brand name the manufacturer assigns to it.

Common combinations of drugs used for breast cancer are Adriamycin, cyclophosphamide, methotrexate, fluorouracil (5-FU), and the taxane drugs Taxol, Taxotere (docetaxel), and Abraxane. Others are Adriamycin and cyclophosphamide and 5-FU (CAF); Xeloda and Taxotere (XT); Adriamycin and cyclophosphamide (AC); and Taxotere, Adriamycin, and Cytoxan (TAC).

Bisphosphonates[15] appear to help prevent cancer recurrences in high-risk women. Studies have been conducted in which randomized trials examined the experiences of women on anti-estrogen treatments who also took a bisphosphonate. Adding the bisphosphonate seemed to help prevent cancer recurrences, and not just in bone.[16,17]

Physicians commonly recommend that women with estrogen-receptor negative tumors be treated with chemotherapy, and also with Herceptin if their tumors contain high levels of HER-2-neu. Common side effects of chemotherapy include hair loss, secondary infections, and suppression of white cell counts in the blood.

If you consider using herbs while on chemotherapy, please do so only after consulting with your medical oncologist.

Individualized Treatment

Chemotherapy often reduces the odds that your cancer will recur. Risk may be cut substantially, but these reductions are not always large ones. But powerful tools now exist to help you consider the possible benefits of chemotherapy versus its side effects. The website adjuvantonline.com provides the Adjuvant service to assist health professionals and patients with early cancer. Often used after surgery, it aids in discussion of the risks and benefits of undergoing additional therapy, usually chemotherapy or hormone therapy, or both.

The software tools at the site help health professionals make several estimates, including: the risk of negative outcome (i.e., cancer-related mortality or relapse) without systemic adjuvant therapy; the reduced risks afforded by therapy; and the risks of side effects of the therapy. Estimates are developed by using information entered about a patient and her tumor or tumors (for example, patient age, tumor size, nodal involvement, and histologic grade). For the best results, an oncology health professional should enter the information into the application.

Genomic assays offer information on your chances of recurrence if you have ER-positive cancer. After surgery for breast cancer, your scores on these assays can help you and your doctor determine whether you need chemotherapy. They can also help you to evaluate the risks and benefits of chemotherapy. With information taken from your tumor, your doctor can offer you treatment targeted to your needs.

In some cases, doctors may recommend that a woman avoid chemotherapy because the woman's breast cancer recurrence risk is low as measured by tests like Oncotype DX, MammaPrint, MammaStrat, and others that probe the genetic nature of individual tumors. Specifically, these tests assist women in making treatment choices if they have early stage breast cancer and are estrogen receptor positive, and if they are estrogen receptor positive, postmenopausal women with a maximum of three cancerous lymph nodes.

The chart below was developed by Susan Love, a former breast surgeon at the University of California at Los Angeles who now heads up the Dr. Susan Love Research Foundation. This chart demonstrates how results of the Oncotype DX genetic assay can influence treatment decisions.[18]

Treatment Options

Molecular type	Hormonal therapy (tamoxifen/ ovarian ablation/ aromatase inhibitor)	Chemotherapy	Herceptin
ER+ and/or PR+, HER-2–(low recurrence score)	Yes	No	No
ER+ and/or PR+, HER-2– (high recurrence score)	*See note.	Yes	No
ER+ and/or PR +/–, HER-2+	Yes	Yes	Yes
ER– and PR–, HER-2+	No	Yes	Yes
ER– and PR–, HER-2–	No	Yes	No

* The original chart says "No" here, but Dr. Harness believes that it should say "Yes."

"For women who are ER positive and/or PR positive and HER-2 negative with high recurrence scores, I would also recommend prescribing anti-hormonal therapy after chemotherapy," Dr. Harness says.

"The Oncotype DX test produces a range of scores; these include a high recurrence score and a low recurrence score," Dr. Harness explains. "In invasive breast cancer, the two really important values of the Oncotype DX are these: We get a number that predicts your chance of having the cancer recur elsewhere in your body over the next ten years. The recurrence score gives us a percentage that we share with you. And because the recurrence score represents a continuum of increasing aggressiveness, the benefit of chemotherapy is associated with high recurrence scores and no chemotherapy benefit is associated with a low recurrence score. Therefore, we get an index, where a recurrence score suggests the potential benefit or lack thereof for chemotherapy.

"The one area for Oncotype DX that falls in between is called the intermediate risk score. A national clinical trial, called 'the TAILORx trial,' enrolled patients with intermediate risk scores into two research arms. In one arm, patients received chemotherapy plus anti-hormonal therapy. In the other arm of the trial, patients only received anti-hormonal therapy.

"Now remember, if you've got a high-risk score, you need chemotherapy as well as anti-estrogen therapy after the chemotherapy. If you've got a low-risk recurrence score, there is no benefit to chemotherapy and you really only need anti-estrogen therapy, whether that is tamoxifen or an aromatase inhibitor. But this gray zone in between the two ranges was the subject of this national prospective clinical trial.

"Unfortunately, it's going to take a while for that data from the study to be reported. But I hope that we find that a continuum exists in the intermediate risk categories, so that as women show higher intermediate risk, maybe we need to make sure that women with these scores get chemotherapy.

"So if you are estrogen receptor positive and lymph node negative, or positive, and are premenopausal with an invasive breast cancer, in my view, you need an Oncotype DX examination. The same is true with the postmenopausal women, and particularly those with one to three lymph nodes containing cancer. We are finding that the Oncotype DX recurrence score is really helpful in determining whether women in that group would benefit from chemotherapy."

Oncotype DX test results may also help patients with ductal carcinoma in situ to decide whether to undergo radiation therapy. The MammaPrint, MammaStrat, and other evolving genomic tests may also help women decide whether to undergo chemotherapy.

"With the Oncotype DX test and other future medical technologies, doctors will gain better insights into the unseen environment of the human breast," Dr. Harness predicts. "As new targeted therapies emerge, the treatment of breast cancer will change. Women who need treatment will hopefully experience fewer side effects, and their therapy will be more effective. Their cancer experience will be guided by treatment maps developed with the aid of genomic analyses of their tumors. Women will have more confidence that they are undergoing the best treatment for them."

Targeted Therapy

Current technology known as immunological or biological therapy identifies garbled messages in breast cells, seeks them out, and targets them. Doctors use powerful substances to select and disable living "software" gone bad inside breast cells. These targeted approaches offer an advance over chemotherapy. Their methods of combating cancer diverge from those of chemotherapy, and their side effects are different and may be less severe.[19]

Chemotherapy does not distinguish between normal cells and cancerous ones. It aims to kill all fast-growing cells in the body, and in its race to find rapidly multiplying cancer cells, it also attacks normal cells found in the skin, bone marrow, gastro-intestinal tract, and other organs.

Commonly used targeted therapy for breast cancer includes Herceptin (trastuzumab) and Tykerb (lapatinib) and Perjeta (pertuzumab). In the future, targeted therapies may replace chemotherapy for breast cancer. Their use signals a change in the paradigm for breast cancer treatment.

Susan Love describes this new approach and shows how it differs from the older system. Her chart provides a simple explanation.[20]

Old Clinically Based	New Biologically Based
Theory: Cancer is a mutated cell that progresses to metastatic disease and ultimate death.	Theory: Cancer is a mutated cell in a supportive microenvironment.
Screening Goal: Find all cancers early.	Screening Goal: Find or distinguish clinically relevant tumors.
Treatment Goal: Remove or kill all cancer cells.	Treatment Goal: Reverse and control cancer cells through microenvironment.
Treatment: One-size-fits-all approach based on stage; higher stage, more aggressive therapy.	Treatment: Personalized medicine; targeted therapy.

Because targeted therapies represent an important aspect of the new treatment approach, it's worthwhile to go into more detail about these substances.

Herceptin

Herceptin (trastuzumab) is a monoclonal antibody that adheres to HER-2-neu, a growth-promoting protein found in large quantities on the surface of breast cancer cells in 20 percent of patients. This treatment often helps slow cancer and may trigger the immune system to more effectively attack the tumor. Administered intravenously, this drug is used together with chemotherapy to treat HER-2-neu positive tumors. Taxol is often added to the regimen.

Side effects from Herceptin include chills and fever, nausea, weakness, cough, vomiting, diarrhea, and headache. In a small number of cases, the heart muscle may sustain damage. Heart scans are performed periodically during treatment to monitor the status of the heart muscle.[21]

Tykerb

Tykerb (lapatinib) also attacks the HER-2-neu protein. The drug is often given together with the chemotherapeutic agent Xeloda. This combination is prescribed for women with HER-2 positive cancer in an advanced stage that no longer responds to Herceptin and chemotherapy.

Other Targeted Therapies

Drug researchers are developing and testing other targeted therapies to combat breast cancer. Initial tests have shown some of their approaches are promising. T-DM1 (brand name Kadcyla) offers a "smart bomb" against HER-2-neu breast cancer. Initial tests in 2012 showed that it prolonged women's lives. Just how long the effect lasts remains to be proven. This therapy links Herceptin to a highly toxic substance, emtansine. Milder side effects are reported with T-DM1: Women don't lose their hair, and nausea reportedly isn't debilitating.[22]

"The clinical trial began with patients who are Stage IV— the term that is used for advanced breast cancer—and focused on nearly a thousand patients treated over more than two years with T-DM1," Dr. Harness explains. "This combination of substances—trastuzumab and emtansine—labeled as a smart bomb, is another example of targeted therapies, which is where all treatments for cancer need to go.

"After two years, 65 percent of the women who received T-DM1 were still alive, versus only 47 percent of those who were in the standard therapy group. Now that number is so important and significant that it was very, very close to the point of actually shutting the trial down because this represented a breakthrough. The trial is ongoing, and it may show even longer survival in patients."[23]

In June 2012, the FDA approved the use of the antibody Perjeta (pertuzumab) to treat HER-2 positive women with late-stage breast cancer. The drug targets cells that produce too much of the protein HER-2 and is used in conjunction with other therapy. The FDA approved pertuzumab for use with trastuzumab and docetaxel.

Some research centers tested the use of a combination of Herceptin and Tykerb for women with advanced HER-2 positive cancers. This combination provided a chemotherapy-free option.[24,25]

Ask your doctor to go over the latest findings with you. Many doctors think that targeted therapies represent a brilliant new horizon in breast cancer treatment, and hold out the possibility that oncologists can one day stop the routine use of chemotherapy in other non-HER-2-neu cancers.

As Dr. Harness explains, "The FDA approved T-DM1 in February 2013 so that it is available for clinical use for patients with HER-2-neu positive breast cancers. Remember, these types of tumors make up about 20 percent of all breast cancers. Hopefully the T-DM1 drug, called Kadcyla, will be used in the neoadjuvant setting—in other words, before a woman's cancer reaches a more advanced stage—in order to shrink down HER-2-neu positive cancers. And hopefully it will also be used in the adjunctive setting, after somebody's already been operated upon for HER-2-neu positive breast cancer."

Anti–Hormone Therapies

Physicians also use anti-hormonal therapies to prevent cancer cells from proliferating in the breast and elsewhere in the body. This therapy favorably alters the environment in the breast that feeds the tumor cells.

Normal body processes, however, are also altered by substances that interfere with hormones in the body. When estrogen levels drop, you start to live in a very different body. Menopause often begins, and you no longer enjoy the benefits of estrogen at levels naturally produced by the body, amounts that provide antioxidant and anti-inflammatory properties and may protect the heart. Estrogen also enhances the body's ability to use insulin. This hormone also increases high-density lipoprotein and lowers low-density lipoprotein, which benefits the cardiovascular system.[26]

So why block estrogen or other beneficial hormones? Some breast cancers cannot grow without a supply of estrogen or progesterone. When patients take medications that block the action of estrogen or progesterone, the growth of cancer cells can slow down or cease.

Tumor cells that need these hormones to grow contain receptors on their surface. These tumors are tagged as estrogen-receptor or progesterone-receptor positive tumors; tumors without them are estrogen-receptor or progesterone-receptor negative cancers. The hormones fit into the receptors like a key sliding into a lock. When this key turns, cell division is promoted in the cancer cells. With the hormones, tumors can dot the breast with cancer—that is, tumors grow faster when the hormones are present.

Limiting Estrogen Production

Researchers have found newer treatments that limit the activity of estrogen. A class of drugs known as aromastase inhibitors blocks a natural enzyme that plays a role in the production of estrogen in postmenopausal women. By thwarting this enzyme, the body is weaned from hormones that fuel breast cancer. Women take such medications daily, and they are only used for postmenopausal women.

Approved aromastase inhibitors include Arimidex (anastrazole), Aromasin (exemestane), and Femara (letrozole).

Side effects of treatment include pain in the joints and muscles as well as a loss of calcium from the bones.

Blocking Hormone Receptors

Drugs known as tamoxifen and toremifene, used as daily pills, block estrogen receptors, preventing estrogen from binding to the cell. Without an estrogen supply, a tumor stops growing. Use of tamoxifen for five years reduces breast cancer recurrence for women with ER or PR positive tumors. Tamoxifen also reduces the development of breast cancer in women with a high risk of developing the disease.

Doctors use a drug called toremifene with women with advanced ER positive cancers. Both drugs are taken daily as pills.[27,28]

Eradicating Hormone Receptors

Faslodex is another substance that damages or eradicates hormone receptors found on the cell surfaces. It is used for women who completed menopause and have failed to respond to tamoxifen or toremifene. Estrogen cannot influence a cell that no longer offers an estrogen receptor. Doctors inject the drug once a month.

Ovarian Ablation

Doctors may also surgically remove a woman's ovaries in an effort to eliminate a source of estrogen and progesterone in a patient's body. They may also use a drug called Zoladex to do so chemically.

Compensating for Anti-Hormone Treatment

These treatments produce side effects. Anti-estrogen therapy can trigger symptoms of menopause, including vaginal dryness, sharp changes in menstrual periods, and hot flashes. Your doctor can help you adjust to these changes.

Medication can be given to treat the symptoms of menopause. The antidepressants Effexor (venlafaxine) and Prozac (fluoxetine) can be prescribed to reduce hot flashes, for example.

Aromatase inhibitors can impact how rapidly calcium leaves the bones, which may contribute to the development of osteoporosis. Bones should be checked with density tests to monitor their status.

Tamoxifen promotes the release of estrogen from the ovaries. But it also obstructs estrogen receptors in the breast. In other organs, including the bone and uterus, tamoxifen acts like estrogen. The drug can cause blood clots, and those taking it experience a small increase in their risk for uterine cancer. Physicians should monitor women for these side effects.[29]

Women using medications to block hormones can still get pregnant, and the medications can harm a fetus. Use barrier methods to prevent pregnancy, such as a diaphragm or a condom. Oral contraceptives, injections, or implants that utilize hormones should not be used by patients on anti-estrogen therapy for breast cancer.

Medications can also affect you sexually. Your doctor or someone on your treatment team can help you find ways to remain sexually active during treatment.

Your treatment team can also help with strategies to reduce pain triggered by use of anti-estrogen therapies, although the causes of the pain are still under investigation.

Endnotes

1. Fineberg B. *Breast Cancer Answers*. Decatur: Lenz Books; 2009: 57–87.

2. Love, S, Lindsey, K. *Dr. Susan Love's Breast Book*. 5th ed. Boston: Da Capo Press; 2010: 111–121, 353–359.

3. Kolata G. Cancers Share Gene Patterns, Studies Affirm. Available at nytimes.com/2013/05/02/health/dna-research-points-to-new-insight-into-cancers.html?pagewanted=all&_r=0. Accessed July 31, 2013.

4. Love, S, Lindsey, K. *Dr. Susan Love's Breast Book*. 5th ed. Boston: Da Capo Press; 2010: 111–121, 353–359.

5. Ibid.

6. Fineberg B. *Breast Cancer Answers*. Decatur: Lenz Books; 2009: 57–87.

7. Love, S, Lindsey, K. *Dr. Susan Love's Breast Book*. 5th ed. Boston: Da Capo Press; 2010: 111–121, 353–359.

8. Ibid.

9. Fineberg B. *Breast Cancer Answers*. Decatur: Lenz Books; 2009: 57–87.

10. Ibid.

11. Lucci A, et al. Circulating tumour cells in non-metastatic breast cancer: a prospective study. Lancet 2012; June 6, 2012.

12. Friedenreich CM, et al. Inflammatory marker changes in a yearlong randomized exercise intervention trial among postmenopausal women. Cancer Prev Res 2012 Jan; 5(1):98–108.

13. Ibid.

14. Lucci A, et al. Circulating tumour cells in non-metastatic breast cancer: a prospective study. Lancet 2012; June 6, 2012.

15. Bisphosphonates block osteoclast-mediated bone reabsorption, are used for tumor-associated hypercalcaemia, and reduce bone pain for breast cancer patients.

16. Fineberg B. *Breast Cancer Answers* Decatur: Lenz Books; 2009: 57–87.

17. Brown JE, Coleman RE. The role of bisphosphonates in breast cancer: The present and future role of bisphosphonates in the management of patients with breast cancer. Breast Cancer Res 2002; 4:24–29.

18. Love, S, Shak, S: Breast Cancer 101 Webinar. Available at youtube.com/watch?v=R4_CqJv3oU4&feature=relmfu, youtube.com/watch?v=sNcjkwWOsK4&feature=endscreen&NR=1. Accessed June 19, 2012.

19. Hortobagi, G, et al. Patient education/ Trastuzumab (Herceptin). Patient information sheet used at M.D. Anderson Cancer Center. August 31, 2012; Houston, Texas.

20. Love, S, Shak, S: Breast Cancer 101 Webinar.

21. Marchione, M: Study: 'Smart bomb' drug attacks breast cancer. Available at huffingtonpost.com/huff-wires/20120603/us-med-breast-cancer-drug/. Accessed June 3, 2012.

22. Ibid.

23. Blackwell KL. Overall survival benefit with lapatinib in combination with trastuzumab for patients with human epidermal growth factor receptor 2-positive metastatic breast cancer: final results from the EGF104900 Study. J Clin Oncol 2012 July 20; 30(21):2585-92.

24. Marchione, M: Breast Cancer Treatment: New Drug Combos Help For Early Stages. Available at huffingtonpost.com/2010/12/10/breast-cancer-treatment_n_794915.html. Accessed December 10, 2010.

25. DeVita, Vincent, et al. DeVita, Hellman, and Rosenberg's *Cancer Principles and Practice of Oncology.* Philadelphia: Lippincott, Williams & Wilkins; 2008: 1608.

26. Longo, D, Fauci A, Harrison's *Principles of Internal Medicine.* 18th ed. New York: McGraw Hill; 2013: 51–57.

27. Sawaki M, et al. High-dose toremifene as first-line treatment of metastatic breast cancer resistant to adjuvant aromatase inhibitor: A multicenter phase II study. Oncol Lett 2012 Jan; 3(1):61–65.

28. Tokura H, et al. [A study of the efficacy of high-dose toremifene in advanced and recurrent breast cancer]. Gan To Kagaku Roho 2012 39(7): 1071–3.

29. Love, S, Lindsey, K. *Dr. Susan Love's Breast Book*. 5th ed. Boston: Da Capo Press; 2010: 111–121, 353–359.

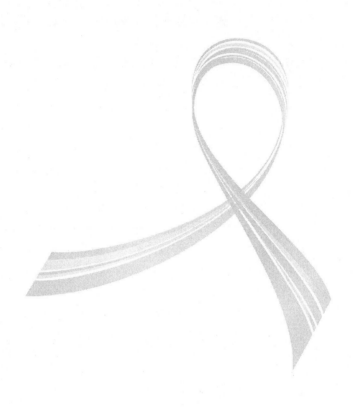

Chapter 8

Radiation Therapy

Specialists in radiation oncology turn to high-energy beams to destroy cancer cells in the breast, near the collarbone, and in the armpit. The beams are similar to the x-rays doctors use to produce images of broken bones and of the chest.

When treating breast cancer, radiation oncologists use rays much more intense than x-rays. These powerful beams compromise the capacity of the cancer cells to develop and multiply. They hit the skin and penetrate below its surface to injure the cancer cells. Sufficiently high exposure to this radiation can kill cancer cells.

For many women, radiation can reduce the chance of breast cancer recurrence by 30 to 70 percent, if administered in the correct dosage. Radiation often helps a woman avoid a recurrence near her surgical scar.[1,2,3]

Women who opt for lumpectomy undergo radiation therapy. This treatment eradicates any cancer cells remaining in the breast, with the goal of preventing recurrence in the breast area. The therapy is considered essential for many women who choose lumpectomy. Radiation also treats large breast tumors, those positioned very close to the chest, and those cancers present in the lymph nodes. In cases of mastectomy, radiation may be used if the tumor was larger than 5 centimeters or if more than three lymph nodes contained cancer.[4]

External Beam Radiation Therapy

When radiation proves appropriate, women commonly receive external beam radiation therapy (EBRT). This therapy, also called whole breast radiation therapy, treats the entire breast and requires weeks of treatment. Radiation oncologists use a linear accelerator to direct rays to the breast area, angling multiple beams.

Accelerated Partial Breast Irradiation

Another approach, called accelerated partial breast irradiation (APBI), administers therapy over a shortened course of time. Therapy is only given to the area where the cancer existed. There are different types of APBI.

IORT

One type of APBI, intraoperative radiation therapy (IORT), is administered to carefully selected patients while they remain on the operating table following lumpectomy—the woman's breast area is still exposed, with the skin splayed back. Two types of IORT are now available at a limited number of centers. One approach gives a woman radiation therapy in a single treatment (single fraction) before she leaves the surgical suite.[5] No further radiation therapy is given. In the second approach, a woman receives a radiation therapy boost to the site of the tumor after it has been removed, which is later followed up with external-beam whole-breast radiation therapy.[6] European women treated this way develop very few new breast cancers. At some centers, carefully selected patients only undergo one IORT treatment, as discussed in Chapter 4.[7]

Dr. Harness suggests that American women get single-fraction IORT treatment at breast cancer centers as part of a research protocol until guidelines for its use are released by American medical groups that follow developments in radiation for breast cancer. (See Appendix.)

Brachytherapy

Some patients qualify for brachytherapy, an APBI procedure that delivers radioactive seeds via a series of hollow, thin tubes dispersed in the breast. These seeds go into the area from which the surgeon removed the tumor. Radiation oncologists repeat this internal radiation outpatient procedure twice a day for five days.[8,9,10]

Other devices can also be used to administer APBI, which is given twice a day for five days (in ten fractions). Each device holds an iridium seed in specific locations inside the device for predetermined spans of time to provide radiation treatment to designated areas. The seed is carefully placed into channels or catheters in a device, held in one location for a calculated, short time period, then withdrawn. At least six hours later, the radiation oncologist reinserts the seed for the same length of time.

Radiation oncologists use three types of single-entry breast APBI devices. They will coordinate with the surgeon to decide which apparatus to use, based on the size and shape of the cavity that remains in the breast after surgery.

Commonly used APBI devices include the Strut Assisted Volume Implant (SAVI), which uses seven to eleven struts or catheters to position an iridium seed to target radiation therapy. Medical personnel expand the struts after inserting the device into the cavity that remains in the breast following the lumpectomy surgery.

A Mammosite balloon can be inserted by medical personnel into a cavity in the breast and inflated. The state-of-the-art Mammosite multi-lumen device provides four catheters through which an iridium seed can move.

Another balloon device, the Contura multi-lumen balloon, provides five paths (catheters) for the iridium seed to traverse inside the balloon. The device's special feature, vacuum ports on either end of the balloon, allows the removal of air or fluid lodged between the balloon and the targeted breast tissue.

Proton Therapy

At a few centers in the U.S., women undergo experimental treatment with proton therapy, but the $100 million cost of equipping a facility to offer such radiation therapy limits its availability.[11,12] Proton therapy claims to provide more precise delivery of radiation to tumors than other types of external beam radiotherapy, and to do less damage to nearby healthy tissue.

Treatment Planning for Beam Radiation Therapy

Radiation oncologists seek to provide the optimal dose of radiation to the breast while doing as little damage as possible to the surrounding tissues. Beam radiation is commonly used to treat women with breast cancer. Doctors use computers to determine the angles of the rays they use. They identify areas of the body at which to aim their beams and mark off the area with ink applied to the skin. The radiation dosage conforms to a plan your treatment team develops.

The radiation oncologist takes time and care to ensure that the position of your body is optimal for the angles of the beams to be used. He or she first simulates a radiation session before starting therapy. Important measurements used to protect your heart and lungs are obtained during this session. A special mold may be made to help position your body for each treatment.

Special external beam radiation therapy (EBRT) technology can improve the therapy you receive.[13,14,15]

3-D Conformal Radiation Therapy

A special treatment strategy, conformal radiation therapy, uses scans to develop a three-dimensional image of the chest area of your body. Having these images allows your radiation oncologist to imagine different ways to administer radiation to you and to choose the best one. The doctor can see the organs near your breasts and reduce the dosage to avoid hitting important organs. At the same time, the doctor can also shape the radiation to the anatomy of the tumor and deliver a higher dosage of radiation to the breast and lymph nodes.[16]

Intensity-Modulated Radiation Therapy (IMRT)

IMRT provides an advanced form of high-precision radiotherapy. The technology allows for more precise radiation dosages. Although the role of IMRT in breast cancer remains limited, it may offer a preferred option in selected patients. IMRT can potentially improve the dose to the target volume while reducing side effects.[17,18]

Preparing for External Radiation Treatment

On the days when you're scheduled for an EBRT session, you should avoid using deodorant that contains aluminum; you can powder with cornstarch instead. Wear soft, cotton clothing to your treatment sessions; this type of clothing soothes your skin. Because you'll be undressing from the waist up and wearing a hospital gown, consider the best outfit to accommodate your clothing changes.

You'll receive radiation treatment in an isolated area where you will be monitored by the treatment team using a camera and a television monitor. The team members see you at all times and stand ready to assist you. You can hear the team members talking to you over a speaker. Follow their instructions on when to remain still and on how to breathe.

If you opt for EBRT, you'll receive it five days a week for four to seven weeks. How soon after surgery you start your radiation therapy depends on whether your treatment plan also calls for chemotherapy. In most cases, patients undergo chemotherapy and then begin treatments with radiation therapy. After patients finish EBRT, the radiation oncologist may administer a "boost" of radiation, using radiation generated by an electron beam.[19,20,21] This boost ranges from five to eight treatments and targets the original location of the woman's tumor. Those patients who are estrogen receptor positive are then prescribed anti-hormonal therapy.

Comparing Therapies

Early studies indicate that accelerated partial breast irradiation (in appropriately selected patients) and external beam therapy produce similar results in eliminating cancer cells in the breast and lowering the risk of cancer recurrence. But intense study of the outcome of this increasingly popular therapy is underway.[22,23]

Benefits of APBI include completing a full course of therapy in five days. Some women may lack access to a nearby radiation center and may be unable to make multiple trips for many weeks to an available radiation center to undergo external beam radiation therapy. With APBI there is a smaller volume of normal breast tissue exposed to radiation, which results in less toxicity to the breast. The APBI option prompts some women to choose lumpectomy with radiation over mastectomy. No long-term data exist regarding APBI outcomes, and many studies are currently evaluating patients treated with APBI.

Choices

Some women in their late sixties and in their seventies who undergo breast-conserving surgery may be able to skip radiation, according to researchers at M.D. Anderson Cancer Center. Anderson Center researchers examined whether 16,092 women age 66 to 79 had needed mastectomy five and ten years after treatment for early breast cancer. The researchers were able to predict whether women in this category eventually needed a mastectomy by analyzing their age, race, tumor size, and estrogen receptor status, as well as whether their lymph nodes were cancerous and whether they underwent radiation therapy. Overall, five- and ten-year survival rates without mastectomy were 98.1 percent and 95.4 percent for those who took radiation and those who did not, respectively.[24,25]

Many women in this category take anti-estrogen therapy if their tumors are estrogen positive.

Oncotype DX for DCIS

In patients with DCIS, the use of the genomic assay Oncotype DX enables doctors to identify some situations for which radiation therapy is not necessary. After breast cancer surgery, women with ductal carcinoma in situ with a low recurrence score on the assay may be able to safely forgo radiation therapy.

These new developments suggest that women should ask their doctors whether they can avoid radiation therapy. "We know it has been an important form of adjunctive therapy for years, and it lowers the chance of cancer coming back in a woman's breast," Dr. Harness says. "But we're now finding out that some women don't need radiation therapy. For example, some women in their 80s may not need it. For those with DCIS, we have a new way to look at it to see if radiation therapy can be avoided. That new test is the Oncotype DX DCIS Score."

Side Effects of External Radiation Therapy

Your body changes with external radiation therapy.

"With external beam radiation therapy, the thing that is so visible is reddening of the skin," Dr. Harness says. "I often tell my patients that they're going to have a really bad day at the beach. By that I mean they're going to develop an irritation that is like a very bad sunburn. Reaction to the radiation varies."

There are also other side effects. "Radiation tends to make the breast firmer," Dr. Harness says. "For some women this is good news; for others, this is disturbing. The breast feels firmer, and the skin thicker.

"If physicians need to extend radiation therapy to the armpit and above the collarbone, doctors worry about lymphedema forming in that arm. In this condition, fluid builds up in the arm and the hand, interfering with normal function. The act of removing lymph nodes and giving radiation therapy drives up the lymphedema incidence to 35 to 40 percent in patients. Patients need close monitoring for signs of lymphedema."(See Chapter 9)

As the radiation treatment progresses, fatigue sets in. The degree of fatigue varies among patients; some experience little, while others become extremely tired.

Mild to moderate exercise sometimes offsets the fatigue. The practice of Qigong may be particularly helpful. This movement therapy comes from China and uses lyrical motions to achieve results. Practitioners of Qigong assert that the practices work with a proposed life energy whose course through the body is stimulated by the artful exercises.[26]

Another study published in 2013 suggests that breast cancer patients have a lower restorative capacity than experienced yoga practitioners.

For women undergoing radiation therapy, depression sometimes presents a challenge. Research conducted in Shanghai in cooperation with M.D. Anderson Cancer Center suggests such patients can use Qigong to combat their depression. Radiation therapy patients who used Qigong during five to six weeks of treatment were less depressed than breast cancer patients who did not.[27]

A randomized trial conducted at the University of South Florida examined eighty-two patients with Stage 0 to III breast cancer who underwent lumpectomy, chemotherapy, and radiation. The forty-one who received six weeks of mindfulness-based training recovered from treatment-related immune suppression faster than those who did not receive the training. Certain T cells were restored more rapidly.[28] Yoga techniques developed by Jon Kabat Zinn were used to instruct these women. Another study published in 2013 suggests that breast cancer patients have a lower restorative capacity than experienced yoga practitioners.[29]

Patients can likely go through radiation therapy while working normal or reduced hours, although some limits on activity may be required. If you limit your activities to those essential for maintaining your life, you can likely go through radiation while working a normal or reduced-hours schedule. It will be important to rest and to sleep.[30]

You may experience breast swelling and tenderness during and after radiation treatment, so adjusting the way you sleep may make you more comfortable. Sleep in loose-fitting cotton clothing in an airy, cool room. Play soft music if this soothes you. Position pillows around you and sleep on your back or on the side opposite the affected breast, if doing so helps.

Cutting back on social activity is advisable if you're very tired, but it is important not to stop all social contact. Social activity satisfies the need for a spiritual dimension in your life.

Telephone friends after an event if you were unable to attend. Doing so preserves a vital social connection, although keeping such phone calls short may help preserve your energy.

Pay attention to interactions and activities that leave you feeling drained of energy. To conserve strength needed for your healing, limit those activities. Consciously choose to communicate more with people who leave you feeling uplifted and who make you laugh.

If you speak with a number of friends frequently, compose short "scripts" to inform them of your progress, because explaining what's going on in great detail can prove tiring for you. Finding humor in your experience helps concerned friends relax.

Skin Changes

Reaction to radiation varies, but after radiation therapy your skin may redden and feel tender and irritable, like you have a bad sunburn.

Use very gentle unscented soap on a washcloth to wash reddened skin, but avoid rubbing and rinsing away markings used for positioning radiation beams for EBRT. Glycerin soap with aloe may prove soothing. Pat yourself dry with a soft cotton towel after bathing.

Soothing creams help the skin heal. Ask your nurse to recommend some for you, but find out if you should avoid using a cream before a radiation treatment.

Soft cotton clothes will provide comfort. Use apparel to protect irradiated skin from the rays of the sun. Loose, high-necked tops with ample sleeves protect reddened skin and can be easy to get on and off. Soft cotton exercise bras help comfortably support the breast. Should your skin crack or blister, ask your nurse for advice on how to care for it.

Considerations

Patients with active lupus, scleroderma, or vasculitis should not undergo EBRT; neither should women who are pregnant. Plan to ask your doctor important questions about radiation therapy.

Questions for Your Radiation Therapist

- Do I need radiation therapy? Which method is better for me, external beam whole breast or accelerated partial breast irradiation?

- What are the benefits and the risks of undergoing radiation therapy?

- If I need radiation therapy, what type or combination of therapies is best for me?

- If I need EBRT, how long should the therapy be?

- Will I need to exercise less while in treatment?

- Is it possible to skip a few treatments?

- Are there certain side effects I should quickly report to the treatment team?

- Is there a difference in the costs of EBRT, brachytherapy, and IORT? What share of these costs must I pay?

Endnotes

1. Fineberg B. *Breast Cancer Answers*. Decatur: Lenz Books, 2009, 46–48.

2. Lange, V. *Be a Survivor - Your Guide to Breast Cancer Treatment*. 5th ed. Los Angeles: SCB Distributors; 2010: 1581-1709 (e-Book).

3. Love, S, Lindsey, K. *Dr. Susan Love's Breast Book*. 5th ed. Boston: Da Capo Press; 2010: 111–121, 326–327.

4. Fineberg B. *Breast Cancer Answers*. Decatur: Lenz Books, 2009, 46–48.

5. Vaidya, JS. Targeted intraoperative radiotherapy versus whole breast radiotherapy for breast cancer (TARGIT A Trial): an international, prospective, randomized, non-inferiority phase 3 trial. Lancet 2010; 376 (July): 91–102.

6. Retisamer R, et al. The Salzburg concept of intraoperative radiotherapy for breast cancer: results and considerations. Int J Cancer 2006; 118(11):2882–2887.

7. Vaidya, JS. Long-term results of targeted intraoperative radiotherapy (TARGIT) boost during breast-conserving surgery. Int J Radiation Oncology Biol Phy 2011; 81: 1091–1097.

8. Fineberg B. *Breast Cancer Answers*. Decatur: Lenz Books, 2009, 46–48.

9. Lange, V. *Be a Survivor - Your Guide to Breast Cancer Treatment*. 5th ed. Los Angeles: SCB Distributors; 2010: 1581-1709 (e-Book).

10. Love, S, Lindsey, K. *Dr. Susan Love's Breast Book*. 5th ed. Boston: Da Capo Press; 2010: 111–121, 326–327.

11. Proton beam therapy holds 'great promise' at a steep cost. Available at healio.com/hematology-oncology/practice-management/news/print/hematology-oncology/%7B37d0ac7d-ef78-4918-9a47-b4e89f55d006%7D/proton-beam-therapy-holds-great-promise-at-a-steep-cost. Accessed April 10, 2013.

12. Breast cancer. Available at protons.com/protons/index.page. Accessed April 10, 2013.

13. Fineberg B. *Breast Cancer Answers*. Decatur: Lenz Books, 2009, 46–48.

14. Lange, V. *Be a Survivor - Your Guide to Breast Cancer Treatment*. 5th ed. Los Angeles: SCB Distributors; 2010: 1581-1709 (e-Book).

15. Love, S, Lindsey, K. *Dr. Susan Love's Breast Book*. 5th ed. Boston: Da Capo Press; 2010: 111–121, 326–327.

16. UMPC website. What is 3D conformal radiation therapy? Available at upmccancercenters.com/radonc/conformal.cfm. Accessed Oct 14, 2012.

17. Lange, V. *Be a Survivor - Your Guide to Breast Cancer Treatment*. 5th ed. Los Angeles: SCB Distributors; 2010: 1581-1709 (e-Book).

18. RadiologyInfo.org website. Intensity-modulated radiation therapy. Available at: http://www.radiologyinfo.org/en/info.cfm?pg=imrt Accessed October 14, 2012.

19. Fineberg B. *Breast Cancer Answers*. Decatur: Lenz Books, 2009, 46–48.

20. Lange, V. Be a Survivor - Your Guide to Breast Cancer Treatment. 5th ed. Los Angeles: SCB Distributors; 2010: 1581-1709 (e-Book).

21. Love, S, Lindsey, K. *Dr. Susan Love's Breast Book*. 5th ed. Boston: Da Capo Press; 2010: 111–121, 326–327.

22. Cortez, MF. Targeted Breast Radiation Linked to Higher Mastectomy Rates in Future. Available at bloomberg.com/news/2011-12-06/partial-breast-radiation-linked-to-higher-mastectomy-rates-later.html. Accessed Dec 6, 2011.

23. Smith BD, Smith GL, Buchholz TA. Brachytherapy vs. whole-breast irradiation: trial by data. Int J Radiat Oncol Biol Phys 2012; July 15; 83(4):1078-80.

24. Albert, JM, et al. Nomogram to predict the benefit of radiation for older patients with breast cancer treated with conservative surgery. J Clin Oncol June 25, 2012. Doi: 10.1200/JCO.2011.41.0076.

25. Albert, JM, et al. Effectiveness of radiation for prevention of mastectomy in older breast cancer patients treated with conservative surgery. Cancer 2012 118(19):4642–51.

26. Chen K, Yeung R. Exploratory studies of Qigong therapy for cancer in China. Integrative Cancer Therapies 2002; Dec 1(4): 345–70.

27. Chen Z, Meng Z, Milbury K, Bei W, Zhang Y, Thornton B, Liao Z, Wei Q, Chen J, Guo X, Liu L, McQuade J, Kirschbaum C, Cohen L. Cancer 2013 May 1:119(9):1690-8. doi: 10.1002/cncr.27904.

28. Lengacher CA, Kip KE, Post-White J, Fitzgerald S, Newton C, Barta M, Jacobsen PB, Shelton MM, Moscoso M, Johnson-Mallard V, Harris E, Loftus L, Cox C, Le N, Goodman M, Djeu J, Widen RH, Bercu BB, Klein TW. Lymphocyte

recovery after breast cancer treatment and mindfulness-based stress reduction (MBSR) therapy. Biol Res Nurs 2013 Jan; 15(1):37-47.

29. Ram A, Banerjee B, Hosakote VS, Rao RM, Nagarathna R. Comparison of lymphocyte apoptotic index and qualitative DNA damage in yoga practitioners and breast cancer patients: A pilot study. Int J Yoga 2013 Jan; 6(1): 20-5. doi: 10.4103/0973-6131.105938.

30. Lange, V. *Be a Survivor - Your Guide to Breast Cancer Treatment*. 5th ed. Los Angeles: SCB Distributors; 2010: 1581–1709 (e-Book).

Chapter 9

Lymphedema: Treating It

After breast surgery your arm may be different, especially if your surgeon removed lymph nodes under the armpit near your breast. These little bean-shaped structures form part of the lymphatic system, which drains lymphatic fluids in the body back into the vascular system. An important part of the immune system, lymph nodes help fight infection.

When these small structures are gone, your arm and your hand may swell. This is called lymphedema. Sometimes the arm does so ever so slightly and you hardly notice it. Wearing a watch on the arm may irritate you. No one needs to tell you to switch the watch to the other arm, or to buy one with an expanding band. It's an intuitive response.

Long after you've healed from surgery, you may sometimes notice a swelling at the top of your armpit after you get out of the shower. It may be gone the next day. Such swelling may go on for years without causing pain or affecting your ability to move your arm—especially if you gently massage the scar tissue under your armpit, do the arm and shoulder exercises your doctor gave you after surgery as directed, perform deep breathing exercises, and maintain a normal weight.

Helping Yourself

You may also forestall problems by stretching your body and your arm with yoga practice.[1] When lifting, evidence suggests that gradually and progressively increasing the weight you bear helps the arm adapt after healing from surgery. Use of weights in an exercise program should be directed by a trained medical team.[2,3] Patients should not exercise with weights or resistance equipment immediately after surgery.

Wearing a compression sleeve while exercising the arm may help you. Donning such a sleeve when flying on an airplane may also assist breast cancer patients, but more evidence is needed to prove this theory.[4]

At all times, avoid putting on jewelry or clothing that is too tight around the hand, arm, and torso. This includes exercise bras that fit like gel. Form-fitting dresses aren't for you.

If you suspect an infection in your arm, treating it promptly is important because infection is a risk factor for lymphedema. Contact your doctor if you experience an episode of cellulitis, an infection of the skin that may manifest as redness, red streaks, swelling, pain, or fever and chills.

Avoid sitting, standing, or crossing your legs for extended periods of time. Avoid saunas, steam baths, and hot tubs. These may injure tissues in your arm. Also avoid use of diuretics, as they worsen lymphedema. Limit salt and caffeine intake, and avoid alcohol.[5,6,7]

All the strategies listed above are used to support the health of your arm and your lymph system. To understand why, consider the engineering of the human body. The lymph nodes that were removed during surgery had previously filtered a fluid called lymph, taking out bacteria and other unwanted material. Under usual circumstances, this lymph fluid flows through lymph vessels as fine as lace, slips through lymph nodes, and pours back into the bloodstream close to the heart.

Sometimes the filtering system doesn't work as well following surgery and radiation. In some cases, a woman's arm may swell considerably. Swelling may begin months or even years after surgery, and the arm can possibly expand to a huge size.

Avoiding and Minimizing Lymphedema

Surgeons are investigating ways of doing surgery that avoid or minimize the development of lymphedema. Other researchers and doctors are also exploring whether lymphedema can be minimized by working with patients early, before the degree of swelling becomes a problem.

Bioelectrical Impedance Spectroscopy

Lymphedema may be more successfully limited if physicians identify it soon after it begins to develop. To do so, doctors can use a small electrical device to obtain a patient's lymphedema index score (L-Dex), which signals the presence of excess lymph fluid building up in an arm. This device, made by ImpediMed, uses bioelectrical impedance technology (spectroscopy) to diagnose lymphedema. In a medical office, both your arms are measured during the period when you visit with your doctor, and multiple scores are obtained. If fluid builds up, electrical signals travel more easily though the affected arm, and comparing that arm against the normal arm can reveal the possible onset of lymphedema.[8] By comparing test results over time, a doctor gains information about the state of an arm at risk for lymphedema, and can diagnose the condition early. The technology is less effective when a woman develops advanced lymphedema.[9]

In his practice, Dr. Harness relies on bioelectrical impedance to help him spot the beginning of lymphedema even before the woman notices her first symptoms and begins taking rings off the hand of the affected arm. These symptoms, when they do appear, include a sensation of heaviness in the arm and slight swelling.

Dr. Harness also uses advanced surgical techniques to help avoid the development of lymphedema.

Early Referral to Physical Therapy

Some treatment teams advocate training patients in physical therapy techniques such as manual massage and compression wrapping immediately after surgery.[10] "This provides patients with tools they can begin using immediately to help bring down noticeable swelling in early stages and hopefully turn it around," Dr. Harness says. "Such instruction is usually given by physical therapists *after* swelling begins. Extra fluid in the arm may be triggering problems with movement and producing pain by the time lymphedema is diagnosed, making it harder to bring lymphedema under control."

Treating Lymphedema with Current Approaches

Current treatment for lymphedema focuses on reducing the swelling and avoiding another increase in fluid. It keeps the condition in check. A popular treatment developed in Germany is now used in Europe and in the United States. Physical therapists usually administer this therapy, referred to as complete decongestive physiotherapy (CDT). CDT focuses on:

- Care of the skin and nails, including the possible use of both topical and systemic antifungal drugs (to eliminate infection of the skin before treatment)

- Manual lymph drainage

- Short-stretch bandaging applied in multiple layers

- Exercise

- Compression garments fitted to the patient, or alternative compression devices

- Lessons on how to manage the condition at home

Undergoing this treatment requires dedicating time to its steps, and medical treatment is costly. Therapists work to achieve two goals: moving an accumulation of protein-dense fluid and breaking down scarring at the armpit.

At the same time, therapists may apply compression bandages, which may be worn twenty-four hours a day for a few weeks. Patients are also measured for and instructed in the use of compression sleeves used to maintain reductions.

A strategy that stretches tissues, known as myofascial release, may be used to help restore mobility in the arm and armpit during CDT therapy. Patients can be trained to perform this therapy at home, but doing so without assistance can be awkward.[11]

When formal therapy ends, patients work to maintain the progress achieved in therapy by wearing compression sleeves during the day and sometimes by wrapping their arms in bandages at night. Effective maintenance is critical to halting the progression of the disorder.

For women with breast cancer, studies show CDT therapy lowers the circumference of an affected arm and the volume of its fluid. Measurements of both circumference and volume should be taken every six months. Compression sleeves should be refitted and replaced every three to six months.

Aggressive use of CDT at early onset of lymphedema offers an important method of addressing this malady and may improve your quality of life. Daily attention to your arm yields important benefits.

Acupressure

At Memorial Sloan Kettering, Cancer Center in New York City, a trained acupuncturist is using acupressure to assist women with lymphedema. She uses the technique in quadrants of the body outside the area of the breast and armpit treated for cancer. Such work may also provide another avenue of help for you when used as a complement to CDT therapy.[12]

Axillary Reverse Mapping

Researchers are trying to find ways to avoid lymphedema. Among other preventive options being examined is axillary reverse mapping (ARM), a surgical strategy that traces where lymph flows through the breast affected by cancer and where it moves through the arm. The goal is to preserve lymph channels and nodes in the axilla (armpit) that drain lymph from the arm, hopefully preventing lymphedema in the process. Surgeons attempt to save these special nodes at the time they are removing other cancerous lymph nodes.[13,14,15] The challenge is to save these structures without also leaving cancer behind.

Other strategies include liposuction, which removes fat from the arm and may stimulate the development of new lymphatic structures that improve the "plumbing" in the arm. Not all surgeons are enthusiastic about this strategy, however, and some believe it should not be used.

In an important development of great benefit to patients surgeons also use sentinel node biopsies, which can help preserve structures in the axilla, as discussed in Chapter 2. However, many surgeons are limiting the use of SNB to work on no more than four nodes in the armpit of a patient.

Expert surgeons also use lymphatic bypass procedures to assist breast cancer patients. The latter microsurgery connects the lymph system to the veins, but gives mixed results.[16,17] Still other surgeons have experimented with inserting shunts in the arm to move lymph fluid, but this technique remains experimental.

Many of these approaches positively impact the arm because lymphedema is thought to arise if:

- The lymph system and its channels are disturbed during surgery

- The axilla is treated with post-operative radiation therapy

- Scars develop in the armpit, helping to block important drain points in the arm

When blockages occur, tissues in the arm become backed up with lymph fluid, which contains protein. Left untreated, lymphedema can become a chronic condition. Much remains to be understood about the lymphatic system and about the lymphedema that develops after breast cancer surgery. But one thing is clear: when more intensive surgery for breast cancer was routinely done, the incidence of lymphedema was higher among breast cancer patients.

Use of Sentinel Node Biopsy Decreases Lymphedema

Fortunately, the increasing use of sentinel node biopsy appears to decrease the chances of patients developing lymphedema. Studies show that lymphedema develops in 5 to 9 percent of patients who undergo sentinel node biopsies, compared with up to 40 percent who undergo full axillary dissection.[18,19]

Between 30 and 50 percent of breast cancer patients undergoing both full node dissection under the arm and radiation may develop lymphedema.[20]

In an attempt to forestall the accumulation of lymph fluid and obstacles to its flow, medical teams use advanced techniques to administer radiation therapy. They also minimize the degree of lymph node dissections.

Professionals also usually caution women about caring for their hands and arms after surgery. Take this advice seriously. Ask your treatment team about moisturizing your arm if you don't receive instructions about this.

Shining Light on Lymphedema

A few centers are experimenting with infrared light therapy to treat lymphedema. This treatment is most effective if administered in the early stages of lymphedema. Use of the light appears to speed healing of wound tissue. Others are experimenting with the use of low-level laser light to combat lymphedema.[21]

In a three-year study conducted in Australia, researchers found that ten women with breast cancer treated for arm lymphedema benefitted from use of low-level laser therapy. The circumference of their arms shrank and remained lower for thirty or more months. These women, who all had undergone radical mastectomy and radiation, received sixteen laser treatments over ten weeks. They experienced a reduction in fluid volume and arm size, and a softening of their skin (except in the upper arm). Patients also reported that pain in their arms decreased. Over time, however, some patients reported that other subjective problems with their arms had returned.[22]

In a study that followed forty-seven Turkish women for twelve months, researchers compared the experience of lymphedema patients (post mastectomy) who received two hours of pneumatic compression therapy in twenty treatment sessions over four weeks, and compared their experience to that of women given twenty minutes of laser therapy three times a week for four weeks. Both groups were encouraged to do limb exercises. Arm volume decreased in both groups, but soon after treatment and at twelve months, the reduction for women treated with laser therapy was more significant.[23]

Stimulating Growth of Structures

New research raises the possibility that retinol (9-cis retinoic acid) may be helpful in regenerating parts of the lymph system in lymphedema triggered by medical treatment. In mice, use of this vitamin A component appears to stimulate the development of new blood vessels in the lymph system and regeneration of lymph structures. Researchers will need to establish that this phenomenon also occurs in humans.[24]

Other researchers are exploring whether other "growth factors" might encourage the growth of lymphatic vessels and forestall or ameliorate lymphedema.[25,26] Still others are exploring whether gene therapy can trigger the development of new structures in a woman's arm (lymphangioles).[27,28]

At multiple centers in the U.S., other researchers are exploring the possibility of using hyperbaric oxygen chambers to assist women with lymphedema.[29] They ponder whether a technology that speeds healing of wounds can help breast cancer patients with their arms.[30,31]

Know the Signs and Stages of Lymphedema

While the researchers work, be vigilant. If you notice swelling in an arm near the location of your breast surgery, be proactive. Find a center that provides lymphedema treatment or go to a doctor or physical therapist trained to treat lymphedema. You can find a center near you by contacting the National Lymphedema Network (lymphnet.org).

Keep in mind that lymphedema develops progressively. In the beginning stage, surgery triggers a reduction in the capacity of the arm to move lymph fluid, but the arm doesn't swell. Without unusual stress on the arm, the lymphedema doesn't cause a problem. Stressors that can worsen the condition may include going out in extreme heat, lifting heavy objects, and performing strenuous tasks too soon after surgery.

Any soft swelling that does develop in this first stage can usually be reversed. Swelling can be reduced by elevating the arm above the level of the heart. With attention to the slight lymphedema, the skin retains its normal structure.

When lymphedema progresses to the second stage, it often cannot be reversed even with more intense interventions. Changes occur in the tissues of the arm that create a feeling of hardness in the arm. Frequent infections may occur, worsening the condition. In the advanced and final stage of lymphedema, the arm becomes greatly enlarged. Large increases in lymph fluid develop, as well as changes in the texture of the skin of the arm. Deep folds of skin may form.

In general, the early signs and symptoms of lymphedema include a feeling of heaviness or aching in the arm, or increased pain and tightness. The arm may tire more quickly than usual.

Endnotes

1. Kollak, I, Utz-Billing, I. *Yoga and Breast Cancer.* New York: Demos Medical Publishing; 2011.

2. Brown JC, Troxel AB, Schmitz KH. Safety of weightlifting among women with or at risk for breast cancer-related lymphedema: musculoskeletal injuries and health care use in a weightlifting rehabilitation trial. Oncologist 2012; Jul 2.

3. Schmitz KH, et al. Weight lifting for women with breast cancer-related lymphedema: a randomized trial. JAMA 2010; 304(24): 2699–705.

4. Graham PH. Compression prophylaxis may increase the potential for flight-associated lymphedema after breast cancer treatment. Breast 2002; 11(1): 66–71.

5. Burt J, White, G. *Lymphedema.* 2nd ed. Alameda: Hunter House, Inc.; 2005: 56, 92–95.

6. Connor S, Connor WE. *The New American Diet Cookbook.* New York: Simon and Schuster; 1997.

7. Wang Y, et al. Current views on the function of the lymphatic vasculature in health and disease. Genes and Development 2010; 24:2115–2126.

8. Ridner SH, Dietrich MS. Bioelectrical impedance for detecting upper limb lymphedema in non-laboratory settings. Lymphol Res Bio 2009; 7(1):11–15.

9. Wang Y, et al. Current views on the function of the lymphatic vasculature in health and disease. Genes and Development 2010; 24:2115–2126

10. Love, S, Lindsey, K. *Dr. Susan Love's Breast Book.* 5th ed. Boston: Da Capo Press; 2010: 437–442.

11. Burt J, White, G. *Lymphedema.* 2nd ed. Alameda: Hunter House, Inc.; 2005: 56, 92–95.

12. Fish D. *Acupuncture and Cancer Care.* Available at community. breastcancer. org/blog/acupuncture-and-cancer-care/. Accessed Oct 16, 2012.

13. Khan S. Axillary reverse mapping to prevent lymphedema after breast cancer surgery: defining the limits of the concept. JCO 2009; 27(33):5494–5496.

14. Bedrosian I, et al. A phase I study to assess the feasibility and oncologic safety of axillary reverse mapping in breast cancer patients. Cancer 2010; 116(11):2543–8.

15. Klimberg VS. A new concept toward the prevention of lymphedema: axillary reverse mapping. J Surg Oncol 2008; 97(7): 563–4.

16. Campisi C, Eretta C, Pertile D, et al. Microsurgery for treatment of peripheral lymphedema: long-term outcome and future perspectives. Microsurgery 2007; 27 (4): 333–338.

17. Tunkel RS, Lachmann E. Lymphedema of the limb. An overview of treatment options. Postgrad Med 1998; 104: 131.

18. Klimberg VS. A new concept toward the prevention of lymphedema: axillary reverse mapping. J Surg Oncol 2008; 97(7): 563–4.

19. Lawenda BD, Mondry TE, Johnstone PA. Lymphedema: a primer on the identification and management of a chronic condition in oncologic treatment. So Ca Cancer J Clin 2009; 59(1): 8.

20. Fish D. Acupuncture and Cancer Care. Available at community. breastcancer.org/blog/acupuncture-and-cancer-care/. Accessed Oct 16, 2012

21. Galanzha EI, Tuchin VV, Zharov BP. Optical monitoring of microlymphatic disturbances during experimental lymphedema. Lymphat Res Biol 2007; 5(1):11–27.

22. Piller, NB, Thelander A. Treatment of chronic postmastectomy lymphedema with low level laser therapy: a 2.5 year follow-up. Lymphology 1998 31(2).

23. Kozanoglu E. Efficacy of pneumatic compression and low-level laser therapy in the treatment of postmastectomy lymphedema: a randomized controlled trial. Clin Rehab 2009; 23:117-124.

24. Choi I, et al. 9-Cis retinoic acid promotes lymphangiogenesis and enhances lymphatic vessel regeneration therapeutic implications of 9-Cis retinoic acid for secondary lymphedema. Circulation 2012; 125: 872-882

25. Guillermo O, Detmar M. The rediscovery of the lymphatic system: old and new insights into the development and biological function of the lymphatic vasculature. Genes Dev 2000 Apr 1; 16(7):773–83.

26. Baker A, et al. Experimental assessment of pro-lymphangiogenic growth factors in the treatment of post-surgical lymphedema following lymphadenectomy, Breast Cancer Research 2010 12:R70.

27. Ibid.

28. Karkkainen M.J., et al. A model for gene therapy of human hereditary lymphedema. Proc Natl Acad Sci 2001.98:12677–12682.

29. Teas J, et al. Can hyperbaric oxygen therapy reduce treatment-related lymphedema? J Womens Health 2004; 13(9):1008–115.

30. Karkkainen M.J., et al. A model for gene therapy of human hereditary lymphedema. Proc Natl Acad Sci 2001.98:12677–12682.

31. Pritchard J. Double-blind randomized phase II study of hyperbaric oxygen therapy in patients with radiation induced brachial plexopathy. Radiation Oncol 2001; 58(3):279–286.

Chapter 10

Paths Through Treatment

*B*reast cancer patients want to trust their bodies again. They yearn to find confidence and comfort in their physical frame, even though their living container has produced at least one tumor. The mass that emerged kept growing until it was detected, escaping the immune defenses the body uses to kill tumors in their early stages. Now the challenge is to eradicate the existing tumor and keep others from arising and growing.

If the patient hopes to live, the disease must be resisted. Medical teams offer tremendous skill in destroying many types of breast cancer with conventional medical treatment. With reverence for the person who is ill, the team often spends months using its vast knowledge and human effort to treat the disease.

The team continuously learns about cancer and its treatment, which improves its skills. Team members share their knowledge with you, often giving you critically important patient handouts. Many patients invest time in learning how to help themselves. This mutual seeking after knowledge assists everyone.

While in treatment, patients know they can help rid themselves of cancer with a heart-healthy diet, exercise, and their own spirit. Movement lowers inflammation, a process believed to fuel cancer.[1]

A patient's grit helps her endure. Reaching out strengthens her connection to others and helps her survive. Some patients affirm the unity of mankind and take the intensely personal step of asking for prayers and good wishes while in treatment. Others affirm the "oneness" of mankind without seeking prayers. Still others turn to their own inner and outer resources. Both types of patients often make new friends and treasure old ones.

Researchers have discovered that patients with a highly supportive network of relationships live longer than women who are very much alone. Women with breast cancer who isolate themselves socially have a higher risk of death.[2]

Complementary Therapies

Many complementary therapies exist that can aid breast cancer patients. "These may help optimize the body," Dr. Harness says. For example, patients may use visualizations in an attempt to help reduce their tumors during treatment. In one mental image, a tiger may gently lick away a tumor. Many patients read inspirational daily affirmations to lift their spirits and support their immune systems as they take chemotherapy and radiation.[3]

Some patients turn to trained acupuncture specialists to help them with a range of treatment-related symptoms, including nausea and vomiting. Acupuncturists often utilize needles, heat, or pressure on certain areas of the skin to induce a change in the body. A Chinese practice used for thousands of years, acupuncture theoretically exploits Chi, said to be a vital energy that runs along paths of meridians in the human body.

Studies show that acupuncture helps with cancer pain, including the joint and muscle discomfort some patients experience when taking aromatase inhibitors. Even hot flashes can sometimes respond to acupuncture treatments.[4]

Why acupuncture works is no longer so mysterious. The use of acupuncture may trigger responses in several areas of the body, including the pituitary gland, nerve cells, and even sections of the brain. These treatments affect immune system functioning and stimulate the release of natural painkillers. Some cancer patients experience less fatigue after acupuncture treatments.

Acupuncture is not the only practice that manipulates the theoretical Chi energy, also known as Qi or Prana. Tai Chi, and Qigong movement, and visual exercises from China, and Kundalini yoga exercises from India are said to raise this allegedly healing Chi. Some women perform Chi practices such as

Kundalini yoga daily in hopes of improving their health during treatment, even though Western science long has denied the existence of this Chi energy.

Demanding physical exercise can be challenging for women undergoing treatment, so the "mindful exercises" of Tai Chi, Qigong, and yoga are more suited to meeting their needs for movement. Of all these Chi-raising approaches, Western scientists now know more about the impact of yoga on women with breast cancer. Studies show that different types of yoga improve anxiety, depression, distress, sleep, and post-chemotherapy nausea and vomiting.[5]

Breast cancer patients using Kundalini yoga may experience increased energy. In a study conducted by the University of California at Los Angeles, one common Kundalini practice (Kirtan Kriya) was shown to improve stress-related aging of cells by increasing telomerase activity in a group of patients who did not have cancer. These activities impact telomeres that safeguard the integrity of our DNA. The telomeres protect the ends of our chromosomes from damage that can contribute to the development of cancer. Telomere activity is implicated in over 60 percent of all human cancers.[6,7,8]

An Australian trial showed that breast cancer survivors who did Qigong exercises in a special medical program for ten weeks showed improvements in perceived cognitive functioning and quality of life.[9] More research on anti-cancer strategies will reveal the best ways patients can participate in the process of healing from cancer while they undergo conventional medical treatment.

Herbs and supplements should not be used during treatment without the advice of your oncologist, due to the possibility they could interfere with chemotherapeutic agents.

Endnotes

1. Friedenreich CM, et al. Inflammatory marker changes in a yearlong randomized exercise intervention trial among postmenopausal women. Cancer Prev Res 2012 Jan; 5(1):98–108.

2. Kroenke CH, et al. Social networks, social support, and burden in relationships, and mortality after breast cancer diagnosis in the Life After Breast Cancer Epidemiology (LACE) Study. Breast Cancer Res Treat. 2013 Jan; 137(1):261–71. doi: 10.1007/s10549-012-2253-8. Epub 2012 Nov 10.

3. Targ EF, Levine EG. The efficacy of a mind-body-spirit group for women with breast cancer: a randomized controlled trial. Gen Hosp Psychiatry 2002 Jul-Aug; 24(4):238–48.

4. National Cancer Institute. Questions and answers about acupuncture. Available at cancer.gov/cancertopics/pdq/cam/acupuncture /patient/ Page2#Section_53. Accessed Dec 31, 2012.

5. Stan DL. The evolution of mindfulness-based physical interventions in breast cancer survivors. Evid Based Complement Alternative Med 2012:758641. Epub 2012 Sep 11.

6. Black DS, Cole SW, Irwin MR, Breen E, St Cyr NM, Nazarian N, Khalsa DS, Lavretsky H. Yogic meditation reverses NF-κB and IRF-related transcriptome dynamics in leukocytes of family dementia caregivers in a randomized controlled trial. Psychoneuroimmunology 2012 Jul 13. [Epub ahead of print]

7. Lavretsky H, et al. A pilot study of yogic meditation for family dementia caregivers with depressive symptoms: effects on mental health, cognition, and telomerase activity. Int J Geriatric Psychiatry 2013 Jan; 28(1):57-65. doi: 10.1002/gps.3790. Epub 2012 Mar 11.

8. Chopra D. Physical well-being, emotional healing. Available at youtube. com/watch?v=_gJN7I0a9XU&NR=1. Accessed Jan 20, 2013.

9. Oh B. Effect of medical Qigong on cognitive function, quality of life, and a biomarker of inflammation in cancer patients: a randomized controlled trial. Support Care Cancer 2011 Jun 19. [Epub ahead of print]

Chapter 11

Survivorship

*I*n modern medicine, doctors define the point at which they complete a medical treatment as a patient's therapeutic *endpoint*. The endpoint defines when the right amount of beneficial treatment has been delivered. More therapy won't help after this point.

Depending on the type of breast cancer you confront, your treatment endpoints are different from those of other women with the disease. As a newly diagnosed patient, you may have several endpoints. If your tumor is estrogen receptor positive and HER-2-neu positive, your endpoints may *include* surgery and recovery, a final round of chemotherapy, and the targeted therapy Herceptin, possible radiation therapy, and a final dose of anti-hormonal medication. If your tumor is HER-2-neu negative and estrogen receptor positive and you're found to have a low recurrence score on the Oncotype DX test, your end points may be surgery and recovery, possible radiation therapy, and anti-hormonal therapy.

All the medical intervention you receive up until you reach the endpoints of your systemic treatment lowers the amount of remaining cancer in your body and hopefully eradicates it. If you are a newly diagnosed patient, an oncologist may be able to declare that cancer can no longer be detected in your body at the end of systemic treatment. He or she then states that there is no evidence of disease (NED). You survive … but for how long, and how well?[1,2,3]

Cancer screenings by your oncologists help monitor your progress against cancer with such tools as conventional blood tests, chest x-rays, and imaging studies. These are often performed by oncologists for as long as five years, but some patients are seen for as long as twenty-five years. The American Society of Clinical Oncology publishes guidelines for how often breast cancer screenings should occur. For women with invasive cancers screenings continue for the rest of their lives.[4] No matter how the affected breast is treated, the unaffected breast must be monitored for life.

When a patient finds it appropriate to go for medical care outside the cancer treatment center, she takes a survivorship care plan her primary care physician can use to continue suitable follow-up care for cancer. In between cancer follow-up visits with their oncologists and surgeons, some women ask themselves whether medical treatment alone ensures a healthy future. Does the body need even more help, they wonder? The answers to these questions are complex.

Some women ponder whether their personal response to their disease should be measured against the severity of their initial diagnosis. Those whose cancers were aggressive or advanced when first discovered may think deeply about such issues. A few others wonder if achieving a pathological complete response (pCR) protects them. This is a response to chemotherapy and targeted therapy that occurs before surgery. In pCR cases, cancer can no longer be found at the main tumor site and lymph nodes in the axilla.[5]

Variable Outcomes

Variability in treatment outcomes adds to the challenge of determining how strongly to battle cancer with personal strategies. That is, for some patients, with a similar cancer and treatment identical to that of long-term survivors, breast cancer recurs in a few years. On the other hand, patients with very serious breast cancers may survive ten years or more after completing rigorous treatment regimens. They survive despite bad initial prognoses that suggested a much shorter lifespan. Some of them achieve such survivals without major changes to their diets or their exercise regimens.

Organization of Medical Care

Why do seemingly similar patients experience very different outcomes? The way different organizations arrange the delivery of medical care may account for some of these differences.

Women survive longer when treated by teams of oncology specialists who care for a lot of breast cancer patients. These teams can be organized informally or they may serve at a breast center. Outcomes apparently improve because of the knowledge, skill, and experience of these oncology teams, which place a premium on close collaboration. In short, specialists talk to each other frequently.[6]

Accreditation and certification efforts in the U.S. and Europe are attempting to ensure that institutions treating breast cancer use practices known to lead to the best outcomes. A study examining the impact of a nationwide German certification program for breast centers concluded that long-term outcomes are better for certified centers with links to oncology experts at institutions like university and district hospitals. Radiologists, pathologists, surgeons, medical oncologists, and radiation oncologists are considered critical members of German multidisciplinary teams, and certified German breast centers voluntarily participate in evaluation of their performance. German law requires that breast cancer care be provided at centers that treat a minimum volume of patients each year.[7]

Improvements in care at German breast centers were linked to:

- Number of treated cases of breast cancer (centralization)

- Annual number of breast cancer operations per center and per surgeon (centralization)

- Use of multidisciplinary teams to provide care
- Establishing breast cancer diagnoses before surgeries, by using tissue samples from needle biopsies
- Providing anti-hormone therapies to breast patients with hormone sensitive tumors, according to guidelines
- Providing chemotherapy to women with breast cancer, according to guidelines
- Providing radiation therapy after breast-conserving therapy
- Delivering radiation therapy to breast cancer patients after mastectomies

In the U.S., quality is promoted by the American College of Surgeons (ACS)[8], which administers the National Accreditation Program for Breast Centers (NAPBC), a program that has accredited 550 American breast centers that meet certain treatment standards.

Certified centers must ensure that:

- All physicians are board certified, or working toward certification
- Nurses show specialized knowledge and training in breast cancer
- Patient care is delivered by a multidisciplinary team
- Centers meet other criteria, including collecting data on indicators of good care

ACS lists accredited centers.[9]

The American College of Radiology encourages best-known practices for *diagnosing* breast cancer. The college accredits imaging programs used to diagnose the disease. These include programs for digital mammography, computed tomography, breast MRI, positron emission tomography, stereotactic breast biopsy, ultrasound, and nuclear medicine.[10]

Genetic Mistakes

Organization of medical care alone does not account for all variability in outcomes. New genetic analyses of breast tumors also suggest reasons for differences in outcomes for breast cancer patients. A 2012 study by the International Cancer Atlas Group took tumor and DNA samples from 825 breast cancer patients. An analysis showed that 30,000 genetic mutations occurred in 810 breast tumors that the researchers had examined closely.[11]

Researchers showed that only three genes were mutated in 10 percent or more of all breast cancers. One of those genes, TP53 (also called P53), is designed to help correct genetic mistakes in cells, but it fails to function correctly in four major types of breast cancer.[12]

Such large numbers of mutations could help explain differences in response to treatment. "There are highly variable outcomes for patients treated with the same regimen and given the same breast cancer diagnosis," Dr. Harness says. "Variations in outcome occur even when women with the same diagnosis fall into different stages of their disease." Some women with a Stage III tumor live longer than women grouped in Stage I. "The individual biology of a patient's tumor can make an enormous difference in treatment outcome. Stage is only a rough predictor of outcome; it doesn't tell us what an individual's response is going to be."

Future Technology

In the future, new technology may help women track their cancers and improve outcomes if cancer recurs. Experimental tests being studied in women with advanced breast cancer may find cancer very, very early. Working at Baltimore's Johns Hopkins Kimmel Cancer Center, researchers are analyzing DNA in cells whose presence signals doctors that cancer may exist in the body.[13] Such cells might form into tiny clusters (from micrometastases) that can grow into a tumor. Researchers have made progress toward early diagnosis of recurrence for women with advanced breast cancer, and they hope to succeed for women with early breast cancer.

Other researchers are examining how breast cancer patients respond to cancer drugs based on differences in the women's genes.[14]

While medical science searches for answers, patients can choose from a number of strategies to guard against recurrence.

SURVIVORSHIP CARE PLAN

After cancer treatment ends, work with your oncologist to develop a Survivorship Care Plan. This wellness plan helps ensure that you receive the best health care in the future. It lists information about your medical history. File a copy of your plan away, and give a copy to each of your current and future primary care doctors.

The plan should include:

- past health problems; diagnoses, treatments and outcomes;

- summary of cancer treatment, with dates, information about effects of cancer treatments, and outcomes;

- a health care follow-up plan with suggestions;

- and a schedule for future examinations, screenings and medical tests.

The NAPBC supports issuing such plans, and accredited cancer centers are asked to prepare them.

Personal Response to Breast Cancer

At the most primal level, the pursuit of survival pushes a woman to define the endpoints for her personal response to breast cancer. For some women, the end of conventional cancer treatment signals completion of the medical response and their own personal response to the cancer. Such women may quickly move on to other considerations such as going back to work, developing a financial recovery strategy, identifying who will provide emotional support, selecting where to obtain spiritual support, and ensuring that a primary care doctor is prepared to help follow up on such post-cancer care needs as pap smears and colonoscopies.

Other women choose endpoints with greater challenges. These women do not consider their struggles with cancer to have ended until they have overcome pain, fatigue, side effects, and the disease itself. Their efforts form part of their attempts at emotional reconstruction. For example, they find out where to obtain rehabilitative care that helps them overcome the challenges arising both from the cancer itself and from the treatment that knocked back their disease. They don't immediately settle for a new normal.

OPTIMIZE HEALTH

Talk with your physician about optimizing your health. He or she may suggest that you:

- Keep physically active and lower harmful stress

- Eat healthy foods, with a balance of good proteins and healthy carbohydrates

- Consume healthy fats

- Keep your weight low and strive for a normal weight after treatment ends

- Avoid tobacco products and alcohol

- Get regular medical and dental care

- Minimize skin and eye exposure to ultraviolet radiation from such sources as the sun and sunlamps

- Avoid contact with asbestos and certain chemicals

After treatment, inform your health care team about issues, including pain or possible symptoms of recurrence. Ask for referrals for help with physical, emotional and daily issues.

Rehabilitation

Harvard Medical School assistant professor Julie Silver, MD, a breast cancer survivor, inspires the latter group to seek physical assistance.[15] In Boston, she provides rehabilitative medical services to survivors and runs a business teaching others to deliver these services. After allopathic cancer treatments end, Dr. Silver works to help patients heal faster, to achieve better outcomes, and to emerge from treatment as strong and whole as possible. In her book, *You Can Heal Yourself*, Dr. Silver explains the possibilities for a healing that focuses on the quality of the life being lived.

Among her tips:

- Don't stay too cool or too hot—you'll get fatigued.

- Poor sleep increases the degree of pain you experience.

- Try to get adequate sleep.

- Pain is sometimes best treated with a combination of treatments.

- Being connected with special people in our lives aids in physical healing: physical changes occur that contribute to our healing.

- New, severe pain in the abdomen, chest, or head should be investigated if the cause is unknown.

- Exercise may alleviate some pain, but avoid activities that trigger pain in the part of the body that's hurting.

Many breast cancer survivors go without formal rehabilitative care but establish endpoints that include daily exercise, which scientists now know lowers recurrence rates.[16] These women also eat a healthy diet that includes good fats. They limit or eliminate alcohol intake, and they quit smoking. They reduce their weight, and if possible, they include weight-bearing exercise in their movement regimens as part of a program to reduce inflammation.[17] They limit bright light at night to maximize the production of the substance melatonin which plays a role in human sleep.[18-24] In short, they work at combating cancer daily.

Mindfulness Practices

Some of these women engage in practices that increase a theoretical body energy known as Chi (see Chapter 10). In doing so, they may continue exercises they used while taking treatment for cancer. As noted in the last chapter, Qigong movement and visual exercises from China, and Kundalini yoga exercises from India, and other practices are said to raise this allegedly healing Chi. Women perform exercises daily in hopes of improving their health. In a study at the University of California at Los Angeles, one common Kundalini practice, (Kirtan Kriya), was shown to reduce inflammation and change the expression of 68 genes[25] (elevated levels of inflammation are thought to play a role in cancer recurrence).[26,27]

A randomized controlled study conducted in Australia showed that breast cancer survivors who did Qigong exercises in a special medical program for ten weeks had lower levels of inflammation in their bodies and experienced improvements in perceived cognitive functioning and quality of life.[28]

Research conducted by M.D. Anderson Cancer Center showed that forty-nine women with breast cancer experienced lower levels of depression when they did Qigong exercise for five to six weeks while they were undergoing radiation therapy. They completed Qigong exercises in five weekly classes. The effect on their mood lasted at least three months after the women exercisers had finished their treatment.[29]

Meditation, repetitive prayer, yoga, and deep breathing all trigger the deep response in the body that Harvard University researchers describe as the "relaxation response" in their studies. At the physiologic level this reaction aids the body in healing. Mental changes occur that assist the patient in positively responding to a disease. Harvard research also shows that all these practices lead some genes to switch on and off. Some of these shifts affect the body's immune system and its inflammatory responses: An important pathway switches off, and turning off this pro-inflammatory factor makes it possible to kill cancer cells. The action may also prevent cancer cells from forming metastases.[30]

Beginning in the 1970s, Chinese nuclear scientists at the Shanghai Institute of Atomic Research performed experiments designed to discover the nature of Chi (or Qi), and reported that it is a form of low-frequency modulated infrared radiation. Some people emit the energy, the scientists said.[31,32,33] Others at the College of Engineering at the National Taiwan University reportedly among those who have also studied Chi as infrared and possibly other forms of energy.

Emotional Healing

For some other women, emotional healing becomes important. They explore potential new endpoints as they seek out ways to heal emotionally from their cancer experience, sometimes facing up to fear of future recurrence. They face their anxiety and depression, and the losses that sometimes accompany breast cancer—such as changes in relationships at work or school; differences in relationships with loved ones, coworkers and friends; a diminished image of the self; a new body image; and a changed body.

They seek encouragement from such role models as Parkinson's disease patient Michael J. Fox. His advice goes a long way toward a woman's emotional reconstruction. When confronted with serious illness, face up to the impact of the disease, but discover those things in life that can still be done. For example, Fox wanted to continue acting but was prevented from auditioning for many parts because of his disability, which causes tremors. Eventually, however, he obtained roles playing characters with Parkinson's. He explained that he found new spaces in his professional life.[34]

Adapt and Expand

Breast cancer support groups also help women deal with emotionally charged issues. Women can often access such groups through social workers at the centers where they are treated.

Many determined patients seek out ways to obtain health insurance coverage and ways to secure or expand personal income. In short, they discover ways to *adapt*. Along the way, they also help their sisters find answers. By adapting and expanding, they apply personal characteristics important to survival.

For example, breast cancer survivors sometimes open small businesses; many people help them do so, including some of their fellow breast cancer survivors. Innovative bankers could help them more. The Grameen Bank, which serves Bangladesh, now operates in the U.S. This bank offers short-term loans to help people of limited means develop businesses that use their unique skills. Such loans can be hard for many breast-cancer patients to obtain through conventional banks. Institutions offering microloan programs like Grameen could be helpful to survivors.[35]

Other women might undergo occupational testing after treatment in an effort to find new roles they can take in the workforce.

Adaptable survivors also educate themselves. Gaining knowledge helps with their emotional reconstruction. For example, women learn about late effects that could occur with the type of cancer treatment they received, and they look for any safe strategies to try to forestall these effects. Among other things, they may learn about treatment side-effects thought to be permanent, such as nerve damage. They search for possible emerging therapies that might mitigate the damage. They consult with their oncologists regarding their findings.[36]

Research Initiatives

Determined women also follow developments that might offer them unexpected solutions. For example, entrepreneur Peter Diamandis plans to finance medical research projects through his X-Prize program.[37,38] The research could address major problems in medicine that block innovation, such as patent laws governing drugs. For example, an open-source system might be created for some much-needed drugs, in the same way that open-source code helped programmers work collectively to create software products like the popular UNIX operating system which is used on some of the advanced computers now teasing out genomic data that has proven the existence of additional types of breast cancer in 2011.[39,40,41]

Diamandis's company, Space Adventures, took tourists to the International Space Station. It also financed breakthrough research that enabled the first privately owned space vehicle to reach suborbital space within two weeks. Diamandis is now following research into long-lived persons, and these explorations might provide insights into cancer prevention.

A few women also know that the U.S. finances an innovative rehabilitation research program designed to bring intense, short-term, advanced research to bear on fields such as orthopedics and immunology used for soldiers. The Defense Advanced Research Projects Agency (DARPA) seeks to help war veterans avoid illness and rapidly recover from injuries. One project would create a universal immune cell to protect soldiers from any deadly pathogen. Cancer survivors might have an interest in such a cell. (Some cancer survivors with other cancers focus on new prosthetics being developed with DARPA money.) A few scientists have suggested that the National Institutes of Health (NIH) should use a similar research model to speed up the development of new strategies to address cancer. A cancer survivor who looks out for herself might advocate for such a program.

At M.D. Anderson Cancer Center, teams of scientists and doctors are assembling for short-term work on specific problems in cancer. One of its "Moon Shot" teams hopes to make breakthroughs in two aggressive forms of breast and ovarian cancer. For breast cancer, the team will focus on triple-negative breast cancer. Its goal: making progress in treatment and prevention of the disease. These scientists also plan to target serious ovarian cancer.

New treatment technology and genetic knowledge will be

used to find promising treatments and move them more quickly into a clinical setting.

The Dr. Susan Love Research Foundation dedicates itself to changing the focus of research to "go beyond a cure to identifying the causes and ways to prevent" breast cancer. The Foundation's projects include recruiting a million women—an "Army of Women"—to participate in breast cancer research initiatives.[42]

Proposals for an NIH ARPA, for medical X-Prizes, for an Army of Women, and for Moon Shots encourage breast cancer survivors who acknowledge their limitations to continue to explore the possibility that their lives can be greatly healed, knowing that if one believes a thing is impossible, then it is. They don't give up. They push the envelope.

Endnotes

1. Titus K. Breast Cancer — Micrometastases turn answers to questions. Available at www.cap.org/apps/cap.portal?_nfpb=true&cntvwrPtlt_actionOverride=%2Fportlets%2FcontentView er%2Fshow&_windowLabel=cntvwrPtlt&cntvwrPtlt%7BactionForm. contentReference%7D=cap_today%2F0510%2F0510b_micrometastases. html&_state=maximized&_pageLabel=cntvwr. Accessed Nov 30, 2012.

2. Fineberg B. *Breast Cancer Answers*. Decatur: Lenz Books; 2009: 81.

3. Perry, MC, et al. *The Chemotherapy Sourcebook*. 5th ed. Philadelphia: Lippincott, Williams & Wilkins, 2012, 1-27.

4. American Society of Clinical Oncology. Breast Cancer Guidelines. Available at asco.org/guidelines/breast-cancer. Accessed July 29, 2013.

5. Kuerer H. Clinical course of breast cancer patients with complete pathologic primary tumor and axillary lymph node response to Doxorubicin-based neoadjuvant chemotherapy. J Clin Oncol 1999; Feb; 17(2):460–69.

6. Wallweiner M, et al. Multidisciplinary breast centers in Germany. Arch Gynecol Obstet 2012; 285:671–1683.

7. Ibid.

8. American College of Surgeons. Many Women Are Unaware of a Key Factor in Breast Cancer Treatment. Available at facs.org/news/napbc1009.html. Accessed November 15, 2012.

9. Ibid.

10. American College of Radiology. Radiation Oncology Practice Accreditation. Available at acr.org/Quality-Safety/Accreditation/RO. Accessed April 2, 2013.

11. Cancer Genome Atlas Network. Comprehensive molecular portraits of human breast tumors. Nature 2012; Oct 4; 490(7418):61–70. doi: 10.1038/nature11412.

12. Ibid.

13. Johns Hopkins scientists pair blood test and gene sequencing to detect cancer. Available at newswise.com/articles/view/596495/?sc=dwhn. Accessed Nov 30, 2012.

14. Szkandera J, et al. Analysis of functional germline polymorphisms for prediction of response to anthracycline-based neoadjuvant chemotherapy in breast cancer. Mol Genet Genomics 2012; Sep; 287(9):755–64. doi: 10.1007/s00438-012-0715-7.

15. Silver, Julie. *You Can Heal Yourself*. New York: St. Martin's Paperbacks, 2012.

16. Ballard-Barbash R, Friedenreich CM, Courneya KS, et al. Physical activity, biomarkers, and disease outcomes in cancer survivors: a systematic Review. J Nat'l Cancer Inst 2012; 104:815.

17. Friedenreich CM, et al. Inflammatory marker changes in a yearlong randomized exercise intervention trial among postmenopausal women. Cancer Prev Res 2012 Jan; 5(1):98-108.

18. Kloog I, Portnov BA, Rennert HS, Haim A. Does the modern urbanized sleeping habitat pose a breast cancer risk? Chronobiol Int 2011; Feb;28(1):76-80. doi: 10.3109/07420528.2010.531490.

19. Hill SM, Blask DE, Xiang S, Yuan L, Mao L, Dauchy RT, Dauchy EM, Frasch T, Duplesis T. Melatonin and associated signaling pathways that control normal breast epithelium and breast cancer. J Mammary Gland Biol

20. Alpert M, et al. Nighttime use of special spectacles or light bulbs that block blue light may reduce the risk of cancer. Med Hypotheses 2009; Sep; 73(3):324-5. doi: 10.1016/j.mehy.2009.02.027. Epub 2009 Apr 16.

21. Bunney WE, et al. Molecular clock genes in man and lower animals: possible implications for circadian abnormalities in depression. Neuropsychopharmacology 2000; 22: 335–245

22. Flynn-Evans EE, Stevens RG, Tabandeh H, Schernhammer ES, Lockley SW. Total visual blindness is protective against breast cancer. Cancer Causes Control 2009; Nov; 20(9):1753-6. doi: 10.1007/s10552-009-9405-0. Epub 2009 Aug 1

23. Sanchez-Barcelo EJ, Mediavilla MD, Alonso-Gonzalez C, Reiter RJ. Melatonin uses in oncology: breast cancer prevention and reduction of the side effects of chemotherapy and radiation. Expert Opin Investig Drugs 2012; Jun; 21(6):819-31. doi: 10.1517/13543784.2012.681045. Epub 2012 Apr 16.

24. Black DS, Cole SW, Irwin MR, Breen E, St Cyr NM, Nazarian N, Khalsa DS, Lavretsky H. Yogic meditation reverses NF-κB and IRF-related transcriptome dynamics in leukocytes of family dementia caregivers in a randomized controlled trial. Psychoneuroimmunology 2012; Jul 13. [Epub ahead of print]

25. Oh B. Effect of medical Qigong on cognitive function, quality of life, and a biomarker of inflammation in cancer patients: a randomized controlled trial. Support Care Cancer. 2011 Jun 19. [Epub ahead of print]

26. Training programs exist for those who teach mindfulness practices. Ask your teacher whether he or she is certified as a yoga therapist. Ask Transcendental Meditation teachers if they have completed a teacher -training program.

27. Chen Z, et al. Qigong improves quality of life in women undergoing radiotherapy for breast cancer. Cancer 2013; 25 Jan doi: 10.1002/cncr.27904

28. Ibid.

29. Bhasin MK, Dusek JA, Chang BH, Joseph MG, Denninger JW, Fricchione GL, Benson H, Libermann TA. Relaxation response induces temporal transcriptome changes in energy metabolism, insulin secretion and inflammatory pathways. PLoS One May 1;8(5):e62817. doi: 10.1371/journal. pone.0062817. Print 2013

30. Healing applications of chi. Available at http://people. howstuffworks. com/chi-kung-exercises7.htm. Accessed November 15, 2012

31. Palmer, David A. *Qigong Fever: Body, Science, and Utopia in China*. New York: Columbia University Press, 2007, 50–53.

32. Interview with Mike Powers. Energy medicines: will east meet west? Available at http://www.mdanderson.org/publications/network/issues/2007-fall/network-fall-2007-energy-medicines-will-east-meet-west-.html. Accessed December 30, 2012.

33. Patient Education Office. *Survivorship: Living With, Through and Beyond Cancer*. Houston: MD Anderson Cancer Center, 2012.

34. Interview with Michael J. Fox [transcript]. Katie television talk show. ABC television. December 26, 2012.33.

35. Yunus M. A short history of Grameen Bank. Available at http://www.grameen-info.org/index.php?option=com_content&task=view&id=19&Itemid=114. Accessed December 20, 2012

36. Latour M. Planning for cancer survivorship. Cure Magazine 2012; Winter. Available at: www.curetoday.com/article/sow/id/2/article_id/2023. Accessed April 1, 2013.

37. Diamandis P. Why we need an X-Prize for drugs. Available at http://www.xprize.org/media-mention/big-pharma-incentives-are-out-of-whack-why-we-need-an-x-prize-for-drugs. Accessed December 30, 2012.

38. Interview with Peter Diamandis. X-Prize program. Available at http://reason.com/blog/2010/04/28/reasontv-peter-diamandis-on-th. Accessed December 30, 2012.

39. Johnson S. Big pharma incentives are out of whack: why we need an X-Prize for drugs. Available at http://www.wired.com/opinion/2012/10/prescription-drug-crisis/. Accessed December 30, 2012.

40. Nikulainen K. Open Source Software: Why is it here and will it stick around? Available at: http://www.law.ed.ac.uk/ahrc/script-ed/docs/opensource.asp Accessed January 4, 2012.

41. Engber, D: I want to be a mad scientist. Available at http://www.slate.com/articles/technology/technology/features/2007/i_want_to_be_a_mad_scientist/i_want_to_be_a_mad_scientist.html Accessed December 22, 2012.

42. Love S. Army of Women—Dr Love on The View. Available at: http://www.youtube.com/watch?v=h1RhTlUdUpk. Accessed October 7, 2013.

Chapter 12

Conclusion

On the day you learn your body has grown a cancerous tumor, life changes forever. Your body changes, and emotionally, you change inside. From that day on, your life journey deepens. Faced with the threat of a disease, you may slow down, freeze, or begin learning at a fast pace.

Some patients become extremely focused after getting a cancer diagnosis. Others go numb. Some patients learn to give themselves time to feel. When the emotional dullness wears off, what's important becomes easier to recognize. This clarity helps you manage your response to the disease.[1]

Clear thinking also fosters the discovery of personal and medical tools to combat breast cancer. You'll be using those tools to survive. In your personal kit, put in a resolution to fight against letting the disease obscure who you are. Find ways to keep expressing and creating. Doing so helps preserve your wholeness. Dynamic people respond to serious diagnoses in inspiring and creative ways that bring meaning to their experience.

Eat your broccoli to combat the cancer, but steam it gently to a glittering green and serve it on a small rectangular white plate like you'd find at a Japanese restaurant. Cooking then becomes an art. Dipping the broccoli in wasabi mustard elevates the art to the realm of science, as the combination creates a killer of some cancer cells.[2]

Pull out the Sunday china for Monday morning breakfast, because every meal is special. You might consider gardening, gathering plants into beautiful designs that celebrate life. Nurturing life pushes back against death.

Some patients share their experiences. So if they want to, let your friends shave their heads in a show of solidarity. Doing so reveals everyone's identity as part of a quiet resistance movement.

What's in your *medical* toolkit depends on the type of breast cancer you have and its genomic nature. Dr. Harness explains: "Fortunately, doctors know more about cancer than they did in the past, and you may be given more than one option for combating your cancer with medical treatments. Because new information about breast cancer is leading to new kinds of treatments, physicians are working hard to help you understand your options. Let your doctors assist in one of the best ways they know how: by helping you make treatment choices."

In the future, more targeted therapies will likely be available to you. To find the best combination of treatments for you, talk candidly with your treatment team. But Dr. Harness advises you to keep in mind that any treatment choices you make will offer both benefits and risks. There are no perfect solutions.

There are more items for your personal list of cancer tools. Many survivors know that expanding your capacity to adapt to changing circumstances helps you, so multiple adaptive talents belong in your personal toolkit.[3]

Finding and nurturing beauty profoundly influences the work of adapting to the reality of cancer. This can include taking photographs, completing needlework, building small items, making wreaths, and doing a host of other activities, including performing or writing music and creating manuscripts. Reflect on your own gifts to find the beauty to express.

Making room in your life to accommodate the effort to resist cancer is an important adaptive tool. It takes effort to eat well, reduce stress, exercise, make changes in behavior, and to take treatment itself. Your organizational skills help you make accommodations.

Along the way, brush up on your skills in fighting fair. This will preserve your humanity against high odds. When conflict arises, measured responses bring people together rather than separating them. In your life as a cancer survivor, unity fosters strength. Find ways to stretch when conflict arises; appropriately communicating what you feel can help. Making space for others to communicate with you also helps.

Triumph

The word *triumph* has many meanings. In the world of breast cancer, the ultimate triumph is coping with your diagnosis, treatments, and survivorship. Triumphant moments may last an hour, a day, a week, or even years. This book provides you with tools, processes, and ideas to triumph over your disease and to achieve your own **Emotional Reconstruction**®

The amazing coauthor of this book, Phyllis Gapen, was an accomplished journalist and a longtime advocate of improving treatment options and finding ways to communicate information to other women with the disease. In 1989, Phyllis was diagnosed with stage III left breast cancer. She lived in Houston, Texas, and all of her care was provided at the world-famous M.D. Anderson Cancer Center. She responded dramatically to neoadjuvant chemotherapy and subsequently underwent breast-conserving surgery.

From the beginning, Phyllis's prognosis was poor. But she dramatically changed her diet, work habits, and stress coping mechanisms. We believe that these changes, along with her excellent multidisciplinary medical care, changed the natural history of her stage III breast cancer.

Sadly, eighteen years after her original treatment, Phyllis's cancer reoccurred in her left armpit. Such reoccurrences typically happen within five years of the original treatment. Phyllis then underwent a second course of chemotherapy, which was difficult, but she handled it with grace. Four years later, Phyllis was diagnosed with stage IV breast cancer. She lived another two years while she worked diligently on our book. We lost Phyllis Gapen on November 25, 2013.

A truly amazing woman, Phyllis practiced what she preaches in our book. She turned a very poor prognosis into twenty-four years of a loving, productive, and compassionate life. Her ultimate *triumph* was sharing her thoughts, processes, and experiences with the world so that others could also triumph.

Thank you, Phyllis, for all of your loving gifts. The world is truly a better place because of you.

Endnotes

1. Conversation with R. Bickel, MD (August 1990).

2. Spicing up broccoli with wasabi or horseradish makes it an even better cancer-buster. Available at dailymail.co.uk/health/article-2036867/Cancer-buster-broccoli-healthier-wasabi-horseradish.html. Accessed Nov 5, 2012.

3. Frenkel, M. Stress reduction (for cancer patients). Available at moshefrenkelmd.com/index.asp?page=2067&inner=2142&lang=eng&textType=long. Accessed Jan 9, 2012.

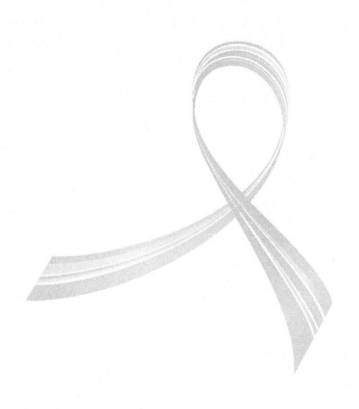

Glossary

Many thanks to Susan G. Komen for the Cure for the use of their glossary.

A

Absolute Risk
A person's chance of developing a certain disease over a certain time period. The absolute risk of a disease is estimated by looking at a large group of people similar in some way (in terms of age, for example) and counting the number of people in this group who develop the disease over the specified time period. For example, if we followed 100,000 women between the ages of 30 and 34 for one year, about 25 would develop breast cancer. This means the one-year absolute risk of breast cancer for a 30- to 34-year-old woman is 25 per 100,000 women (1 per 4,000 women).

Acupuncture
Use of very thin needles inserted at precise points on the body that may help control pain and other side effects of treatment or breast cancer itself. It is a type of integrative or complementary therapy.

Adjuvant (Systemic) Therapy
Treatment given in addition to surgery and radiation to treat breast cancer that may have spread to other parts of the body. It may include chemotherapy, targeted therapy and/or hormone therapy.

Advocacy (see **Breast Cancer Advocacy**)

Alopecia
Hair loss.

Alternative Therapy
Any therapy used instead of standard medical treatments such as surgery, chemotherapy and hormone therapy. Alternative therapies are different from integrative and complementary therapies, which are used in addition to standard treatments. Alternative therapies have not been shown to be effective in treating breast cancer, so it is not safe to use them.

Amenorrhea
The absence or stopping of menstrual periods.

Anesthesia
Loss of feeling or sensation that keeps a person from feeling pain during surgery or other medical procedures. Local or regional anesthesia may be used for a specific part of the body, such as the breast, by injection of a drug into that area. General anesthesia numbs the entire body and puts a person to sleep with drugs that are injected into a vein or inhaled.

Aneuploid (DNA Ploidy)
The presence of an abnormal number of chromosomes in cancer cells.

Angiogenesis
The growth of new blood vessels that cells need to grow.

Antibody
A protein made by white blood cells that is part of the body's immune system. Each antibody binds to a certain antigen (foreign substance, such as bacteria) and helps the body fight the antigen.

Antibody Therapy
A drug containing an antibody that is specially made to target certain cancer cells. See Antibody.

Anti-carcinogen
An agent that counteracts carcinogens (cancer causing agents).

Antiemetic
A medicine that prevents or relieves nausea and vomiting.

Antigen
A substance that causes the body to make an immune response. This immune response often involves making antibodies.

Antioxidant
A substance that protects the body from damage by oxidizing agents. Oxidizing agents are always present in the body and

are often beneficial. However, when large amounts of oxidants are present in cells, they can cause damage, especially to DNA. This can lead to abnormal cell growth. Antioxidants include beta-carotene and vitamins A, C and E.

Apoptosis
A normal cell process in which a genetically programmed series of events leads to the death of a cell. Cancer cells may block apoptosis.

Areola
The darkly shaded circle of skin surrounding the nipple.

Aromatase Inhibitors
Hormone therapy drugs that lower estrogen levels in the body by blocking aromatase, an enzyme that converts other hormones into estrogen. Aromatase inhibitors are used to treat postmenopausal women with hormone-receptor positive breast cancer.

Aspirate
To remove fluid and a small number of cells.

Atrophic Vaginitis (see Vaginal Atrophy)

Atypical Hyperplasia
A benign (not cancer) breast condition where breast cells are growing rapidly (proliferating). The proliferating cells look abnormal under a microscope. Although atypical hyperplasia is not breast cancer, it increases the risk of breast cancer.

Autologous
A blood donation or tissue graft from a person's own body rather than from a donor. For example, autologous breast reconstruction techniques use skin and tissue flaps (grafts) from a person's own body.

Axilla
The underarm area.

Axillary Dissection (Axillary Sampling)
Surgical procedure to remove some or all of the lymph nodes from the underarm area so that the nodes can be examined under a microscope to check whether or not cancer cells are present.

Axillary Lymph Nodes
The lymph nodes in the underarm area.

Ayurveda
An integrative or complementary medical system from India that involves diet, exercise, meditation and massage. Ayurveda means "life-knowledge."

B

Benign
Not cancerous. Does not invade nearby tissue or spread to other parts of the body.

Benign Breast Conditions (Benign Breast Disease)
Noncancerous conditions of the breast that can result in lumps or other abnormalities. Examples include cysts and fibroadenomas.

Benign Phyllodes Tumor
A rare benign (not cancer) breast condition similar to a fibroadenoma. A lump may be felt, but is usually painless.

Bilateral Prophylactic Mastectomy
Surgery where both breasts are removed to prevent breast cancer from developing.

Biobank (Tissue Repository)
A large collection of tissue samples and medical data that is used for research studies.

Bioimpedance (Bioelectrical Impedance Analysis)
A method of measuring the amount of fluid in body tissues.

Biological Therapy
A therapy that targets something specific to the biology of the cancer cell, as opposed to chemotherapy, which attacks all rapidly dividing cells. Often used to describe therapies that use the immune system to fight cancer (immunotherapy). Trastuzumab (Herceptin) is an example of a biological or targeted therapy agent.

Biomarker
A substance found in blood, other body fluids or tissues that can be measured and is a sign of disease or another process in the body (normal or abnormal). It also may be used to see how well the body responds to a treatment for a disease.

Biopsy
Removal of tissue to be tested for cancer cells.

Bisphosphonates
Drugs used to strengthen bones and decrease the rate of bone fractures and pain due to breast cancer metastases to the bone.

Body Mass Index (BMI)
A measure used to estimate body fat. BMI takes into account a person's height and weight. Calculate your BMI.

Bone Scan
A test done to check for signs of cancer in the bones. A small amount of radioactive material is injected into the bloodstream. It collects in the bones, especially abnormal areas, and is detected by a scanner. Bone scans can show cancer as well as benign bone diseases (like arthritis).

Boost
Additional dose of radiation to the part of the breast that had the tumor.

BRCA1/BRCA2 Genes (BReast CAncer genes)
Genes that help limit cell growth. A mutation (change) in one of these genes increases a person's risk of breast, ovarian and certain other cancers.

Brachytherapy
A procedure that uses targeted radiation therapy from inside the tumor bed.

Breast Cancer
An uncontrolled growth of abnormal breast cells.

Breast Cancer Advocacy
Influencing targeted audiences to promote the support of breast cancer issues.

Breast Cancer Survivor (see **Survivor**)

Breast Conserving Surgery (see **Lumpectomy**)

Breast Density
A measure used to describe the relative amounts of fat and tissue in the breasts as seen on a mammogram.

Breast-Specific Gamma Imaging (see **Nuclear Medicine Imaging of the Breast**)

Breast Imaging Reporting and Data System (BI-RADS®)
A system developed by the American College of Radiology to provide a standard way to describe the findings on a mammogram.

Breast Reconstruction
Surgery to restore the look and feel of the breast after mastectomy.

Breast Self-Examination (BSE)

A method that may help women become familiar with the normal look and feel of their breasts. BSE is not recommended as a breast cancer screening tool because it has not been shown to decrease breast cancer death.

Breast Tomosynthesis (3D Digital Mammography, Digital Tomosynthesis)

A tool that uses a digital mammography machine to take multiple two dimensional (2D) X-ray images of the breast. Computer software combines the multiple 2D images into a three dimensional image. Breast tomosynthesis is not a standard breast cancer screening tool at this time.

C

Cachexia

Loss of appetite and weight.

Calcifications

Deposits of calcium in the breast that appear as bright, white spots on a mammogram. Most calcifications are not cancer. However, tight clusters or lines of tiny calcifications (called microcalcifications) can be a sign of breast cancer.

Cancer

General name for over 100 diseases with uncontrolled cell growth.

Cancer Staging (see **Staging**)

Carcinoma in Situ (in Situ Carcinoma)

Condition where abnormal cells are found in the milk ducts or lobules of the breast, but not in the surrounding breast tissue. In situ means "in place." See ductal carcinoma in situ and lobular carcinoma in situ.

Case-Control Study

An observational study that looks at two groups–one with people who already have the outcome of interest (cases), and one with people who do not (controls). For example, the cases may be women with breast cancer and the controls may be cancer-free women. The two groups are then compared to see if any characteristic was more common in the past history of one group compared to the other.

Case Series

A health care provider's observations of a group of patients who are given a certain type of treatment.

Catheter
A small tube used to deliver fluids to (or remove them from) the body.

Centigray (Centigrays)
One centigray describes the amount of radiation absorbed by the body and is equivalent to 1 RAD (radiation absorbed dose).

Chemoprevention
A drug or combination of drugs used to lower the risk of breast cancer in cancer-free women at higher risk.

Chemotherapy
A drug or combination of drugs that kills cancer cells in various ways.

Clinical Breast Examination (CBE)
A physical exam done by a health care provider to check the look and feel of the breasts and underarm for any changes or abnormalities (such as lumps).

Clinical Trials
Research studies that test the benefits of possible new ways to detect, diagnose, treat or prevent disease. People volunteer to take part in these studies.

Cognitive (function)
Mental processes related to understanding, such as reasoning and problem-solving.

Cohort Study
A study that follows a large group of people (a cohort) over time.

Co-Insurance (see **Co-Payment**)

Complementary Therapies (Integrative Therapies)
Therapies (such as acupuncture or massage) used in addition to standard medical treatments. Complementary therapies are not used to treat cancer, but they may help improve quality of life and relieve some side effects of treatment or the cancer itself. When complementary therapies are combined with standard medical care, they are often called integrative therapies.

Computerized Axial Tomography (CAT) Scan (see **CT Scan**)

95% Confidence Interval (95% CI)
A statistical concept that shows there is a 95 percent probability the 'true' measure is found within a range of measures computed from a single study. For example,

if the 95% confidence interval for a survival rate is 75 to 90 percent, there is a 95 percent chance the true survival rate falls between 75 and 90 percent.

Co-Payment (Co-Insurance)
In an insurance plan, the portion of medical costs a person must pay (the portion not covered by his/her insurance policy).

Core Needle Biopsy
A needle biopsy that uses a hollow needle to remove samples of tissue from an abnormal area in the breast.

Co-Survivor
A person who lends support to someone diagnosed with breast cancer, from the time of diagnosis through treatment and beyond. Co-survivors may include family members, spouses or partners, friends, health care providers and colleagues.

CT Scan (Computerized Tomography Scan, Computerized Axial Tomography (CAT) Scan)
A series of pictures created by a computer linked to an X-ray machine. The scan gives detailed internal images of the body.

Cumulative Risk
The sum of a person's chances of developing a disease (like breast cancer) over the course of a lifetime (usually defined as birth up to age 85). For example, the cumulative (lifetime) risk of breast cancer for women is about 1 in 8 (or about 12 percent). This means for every 8 women, one will be diagnosed with breast cancer during her lifetime (up to age 85).

Cyst
A fluid-filled sac.

Cytopathologist
A pathologist who specializes in looking at individual cells. A cytopathologist is needed to interpret the results of fine needle aspiration.

Cytotoxic
Toxic, or deadly, to cells (cell killing). Often used to describe chemotherapy.

D

Deductible (Insurance Deductible)
The pre-set amount of medical costs a person must pay before insurance payments begin.

Definitive Surgery
All of the known tumor is removed and no follow-up surgery is needed.

Diabetic Mastopathy
A rare benign (not cancer) breast condition that consists of small hard masses in the breast. It occurs most often in women with insulin-dependent (type 1) diabetes.

Diagnosis
Identification of a disease from its signs and symptoms.

Diagnostic Mammogram
A mammogram used to check symptoms of breast cancer (such as a lump) or an abnormal finding noted on a screening mammogram or clinical breast exam. It involves two or more X-ray views of the breast.

Diagnostic Radiologist (Radiologist)
A health care provider who specializes in the diagnosis of diseases using X-rays.

Diploid (DNA Ploidy)
The presence of a normal number of chromosomes in cancer cells.

Disease-Free Survival Rate
Percent of people alive and without disease at a certain time (often five years or ten years) after treatment. Those who die from causes other than the disease under study are not included in this measure.

Distant Recurrence (see **Metastases**)

DNA (Deoxyribonucleic Acid)
The information contained in a gene.

Dose-Dense Therapy
Chemotherapy given over a shorter (more condensed) time period compared to standard therapy. The frequency of treatment sessions is increased, so the length of the treatment period is shortened.

Down-Staging
Lowering the stage of a cancer from its original stage (or the stage it was thought to be). Down-staging occurs most often after a good response to neoadjuvant therapy. Neoadjuvant therapy is chemotherapy or hormone therapy used as a first treatment (before surgery) for some large or advanced breast cancers. Neoadjuvant therapy can shrink a tumor such that it lowers the

stage of the breast cancer and a lumpectomy, instead of a mastectomy, can be done.

Duct (Milk Duct, Mammary Duct)
A canal that carries milk from the lobules to a nipple opening during breastfeeding (see figure).

Ductal Carcinoma in Situ (DCIS, Intraductal Carcinoma)
A non-invasive breast cancer that begins in the milk ducts of the breast, but has not invaded nearby breast tissue. Also called stage 0 or pre-invasive breast carcinoma.

Ductal Papilloma (see Intraductal Papilloma)

E

Early Breast Cancer
Cancer that is contained in the breast or has only spread to lymph nodes in the underarm area. This term often describes stage I and stage II breast cancer.

Edema
Excess fluid in body tissues that causes swelling.

Endocrine Manipulation (see Hormone Therapy)

Endometrial Cancer
Cancer of the endometrium (the lining of the uterus).

Enzyme
A protein that speeds up biologic reactions in the body.

Epidemiology
The study of the causes and prevention of disease.

Estradiol
The most biologically active, naturally occurring estrogen in women.

Estrogen
A female hormone produced by the ovaries and adrenal glands that is important to reproduction. Some cancers need estrogen to grow.

Estrogen Receptors
Specific proteins in cells that estrogen hormones attach to. A high number of estrogen receptors on a breast cancer cell often means the cancer cell needs estrogen to grow.

Etiology
The cause(s) of a disease.

Excisional Biopsy
Surgical procedure that removes the entire abnormal area (plus some surrounding normal tissue) from the breast.

External Beam Radiation Therapy (see **Radiation Therapy**)

F

False Negative
A test result that incorrectly reports a person is disease-free when she/he actually has the disease.

False Positive
A test result that incorrectly reports a person has a disease when she/he does not have the disease.

Family History (Family Medical History)
A record of the current and past health conditions of a person's biological (blood-related) family members that may help show a pattern of certain diseases within a family.

Fat Necrosis
A benign (not cancer) breast change in which the breast responds to trauma with a firm, irregular mass, often years after the event. The mass is the result of fatty tissue dying, after either surgery or blunt trauma to the breast. This breast change does not increase risk of breast cancer.

Fibroadenoma
A benign (not cancer) fibrous tumor that may occur at any age, but is more common in young adulthood.

Fibrocystic Condition (Fibrocystic Changes)
A general term used to describe a benign (not cancer) breast condition that may cause painful cysts or lumpy breasts.

Fine Needle Aspiration (FNA, Fine Needle Biopsy)
A biopsy procedure that uses a thin, hollow needle to remove a sample of cells from the abnormal area of the breast.

First-Degree Relative (Immediate Family Member)
A person's mother, father, sister, brother or child.

First-Line Therapy
The initial (first) therapy used in a person's cancer treatment.

Flow Cytometry
A laboratory test done on tumor tissue to measure the growth rate of the cancer cells and to check if the cells have too much DNA.

Fluorescence In Situ Hybridization (FISH)
A laboratory test done on breast tumor tissue to find out the number of copies of the HER2/ neu gene contained in the cancer cells.

Frozen Section
Process where a portion of tissue from a surgical biopsy is frozen so a thin slice can be studied to check for cancer. Frozen section results are only preliminary and always need to be confirmed by other methods.

G

Gail Model (Breast Cancer Risk Assessment Tool)
A tool that uses personal and family history to estimate a woman's risk of invasive breast cancer.

Galactocele
A milk-filled cyst.

Genes
The part of a cell that contains DNA. The DNA information in a person's genes is inherited from both sides of a person's family.

Gene Expression
Process in which a gene gets turned on in a cell to make RNA and proteins.

Gene Expression Profiling (see **Tumor Profiling**)

Gene Mutation
Any change in the DNA (the information contained in a gene) of a cell. Gene mutations can be harmful, beneficial or have no effect.

Gene Variant of Uncertain Significance
A gene mutation not currently known to increase breast cancer risk.

General Practitioner (Internist, Physician)
The personal or family physician who may first find a suspicious area in the breast through a clinical breast exam or mammogram.

Generic
The chemical name of a drug, not the brand name. The chemical formulations of a generic drug and the brand name drug are the same.

Genetic (Hereditary)
Related to genes. The information in a person's genes can be passed on (inherited) from either parent.

Genetic Susceptibility (Genetic Predisposition)
An increased likelihood or chance of developing a disease due to specific changes in a person's genes passed on from either parent.

Genetic Testing
Analyzing DNA to look for a gene mutation that may show an increased risk for developing a specific disease.

Genome
The total genetic information of an organism.

Genomics
The study of genes and their functions.

Glandular Tissue (in the breast)
The tissue in the breast that includes the milk ducts and lobules.

Grade (see **Tumor Grade**)

Guaranteed Renewable Insurance
A health insurance policy that requires the insurance company to renew your policy for a certain amount of time, even if your health condition changes.

H

H&E (Hematoxylin and Eosin) Staining
A laboratory test that gives color to cells so cell structures can be identified.

HER2/neu (Human Epidermal Growth Factor Receptor 2, erbB2)
A protein involved in cell growth and survival that appears on the surface of some breast cancer cells. **HER2/neu-negative** breast cancers have little or no HER2/neu protein. **HER2/neu-positive** breast cancers have a lot of HER2/neu protein. HER2/neu-positive tumors can be treated with the targeted therapy drug trastuzumab (Herceptin).

Herceptin (see **Trastuzumab**)

Hereditary (see **Genetic**)

Homeopathy (Homeopathic Medicine)

A medical system based on a belief that "like cures like." Natural substances are specially prepared in small amounts to restore health. These substances cause symptoms similar to the condition they are meant to treat in healthy people. There are limited data on the safety of these substances.

Hormones

Chemicals made by certain glands and tissues in the body, often in response to signals from the pituitary gland or the adrenal gland. Hormones have specific effects on specific target organs and tissues. Examples include estrogen and progesterone. Hormones can also be made in a laboratory.

Hormone Receptors

Specific proteins on cells that hormones attach to. A high number of hormone receptors on a breast cancer cell often means the cancer cell needs the hormone to grow.

Hormone Receptor Status

Shows whether or not a breast cancer needs hormones to grow. A **hormone receptor-positive** cancer needs hormones to grow. A **hormone receptor-negative** cancer does not need hormones to grow. See Hormone Receptor.

Hormone Replacement Therapy (see **Menopausal Hormone Therapy**)

Hormone Therapy (Endocrine Therapy, Endocrine Manipulation)

Treatment that works by keeping cancer cells with hormone receptors from getting the hormones they need to grow.

Hospice

A philosophy of care focusing on improving quality of life and easing pain and other symptoms at the end stage of a terminal illness. Hospice care also provides support services to patients and their families.

Hyperplasia (Usual and Atypical Hyperplasia)

A benign (not cancer) breast condition where breast cells are growing rapidly (proliferating). Although hyperplasia is not breast cancer, it increases the risk of breast cancer. In usual hyperplasia, the proliferating cells look normal under a microscope. In atypical hyperplasia, the proliferating cells look abnormal.

I

Immediate Family Member (First-Degree Relative)
A person's mother, father, sister, brother or child.

Immunotherapy
Therapies that use the immune system to fight cancer. These therapies target something specific to the biology of the cancer cell, as opposed to chemotherapy, which attacks all rapidly dividing cells. See Biological Therapy.

Immunohistochemistry (IHC)
A laboratory test done on tumor tissue to detect the amount of HER2/neu protein on the surface of the cancer cells.

Implant (Breast Implant)
An "envelope" containing silicone, saline or both, that is used to restore the breast form after a mastectomy (or for other cosmetic reasons).

In Situ
Carcinoma (see **Carcinoma in Situ**)

In-Network Provider
The health care providers and medical centers (hospitals and other treatment centers) that are part of a particular group health plan or health maintenance organization (HMO).

Incidence
The number of new cases of a disease that develop in a specific time period.

Incisional Biopsy
Surgical biopsy that removes only part of the tumor.

Indemnity Policy
A prepayment insurance plan that gives services or a cash payment for medical care needed in times of illness or disability.

Induction Chemotherapy (see **Neoadjuvant Chemotherapy**)

Inflammatory Breast Cancer (IBC)
A rare and aggressive form of invasive breast cancer. Its main symptoms are swelling (inflammation) and redness of the breast. The skin on the breast may look dimpled, like the skin of an orange, and may be warm to the touch.

Informed Consent
The process through which a person learns about the possible benefits and side effects of a treatment plan and then accepts or declines the treatment. The person is usually asked to sign a consent form, but may stop the treatment at any time and get other medical care.

Infraclavicular Lymph Nodes
The lymph nodes below the clavicle (collarbone). See **Lymph Nodes**.

Insurance Payment Cap
A maximum amount an insurance company will pay out in a given time period.

Insurance Premium (Premium)
The cost of insurance coverage for a certain period of time.

Integrative Therapies (see **Complementary Therapies**)

Intraductal
Within the milk duct. Intraductal can describe a benign (not cancerous) or malignant (cancerous) process.

Intraductal Hyperplasia
An excess of cells growing within the milk ducts of the breast.

Intraductal Papilloma (Ductal Papilloma)
Small, benign (not cancer) growths that begin in the ducts of the breast and usually cannot be felt. Symptoms include a bloody or clear nipple discharge.

Intravenous or IV
Being within or entering the body through the veins.

Invasive Breast Cancer
Cancer that has spread from the original location (milk ducts or lobules) into the surrounding breast tissue and possibly into the lymph nodes and other parts of the body. **Invasive ductal cancer** begins in the milk ducts. **Invasive lobular cancer** begins in the lobules of the breast.

Investigational New Drug (New Experimental Treatment)
A chemical or biological drug that has been approved for use by researchers in studies, but is not yet available outside of a clinical trial.

K

Ki-67 Rate
A common way to measure proliferation rate. The more cells the Ki-67 antibody attaches to on

a tissue sample, the more likely the tumor cells are to grow and divide rapidly.

L

Lactation
The process of producing milk and breastfeeding a child.

Large Veins (Deep Veins)
The large veins deep inside the legs that carry blood from the legs back to the heart.

Late-Stage Cancer (see **Metastatic Breast Cancer**)

Lesion
Area of abnormal tissue.

Lifetime Risk
The chance of developing a disease (like breast cancer) over the course of a lifetime (usually defined as birth up to age 85). For example, the lifetime risk of breast cancer for women is 1 in 8 (or about 12 percent). This means for every 8 women, one will be diagnosed with breast cancer during her lifetime (up to age 85).

Linear Accelerator
The device used during radiation therapy to direct X-rays into the body.

Liver Scan
An image of the liver that can show the presence or absence of a tumor.

Lobular Carcinoma in Situ (LCIS, Lobular Neoplasia in Situ)
A condition where abnormal cells grow in the lobules of the breast. LCIS increases the risk of breast cancer.

Lobular Neoplasia in Situ (see **Lobular Carcinoma in Situ**)

Lobules
Ball-shaped sacs in the breast that produce milk.

Local Anesthetic
Anesthesia that only numbs the tissue in a certain area. See Anesthesia.

Local Treatment
Treatment that focuses on getting rid of the cancer from a certain (local) area. In breast cancer, the local area includes the breast, the chest wall and lymph nodes in the underarm area (axillary nodes). Local treatment for breast cancer includes surgery with or without radiation therapy.

Localized Breast Cancer
Cancer that is contained in the breast and has not spread to nearby tissue, lymph nodes or other organs.

Locally Advanced Breast Cancer (Stage III Breast Cancer)
Cancer that has spread beyond the breast to the skin or chest wall, but not to distant organs like the lungs or liver. It also refers to a tumor that is larger than five centimeters (about two inches) in size.

Local Recurrence (Recurrence)
The return of cancer to the same breast or to the same side chest wall.

Lump
Any mass in the breast or elsewhere in the body.

Lumpectomy (Breast Conserving Surgery)
Surgery that removes only part of the breast—the part containing and closely surrounding the tumor.

Lymph Nodes (Lymph Glands)
Small groups of immune cells that act as filters for the lymphatic system. Clusters of lymph nodes are found in the underarms, groin, neck, chest and abdomen.

Lymph Node Status
Shows whether or not cancer has spread to the lymph nodes. **Lymph node-positive** means that cancer has spread to the lymph nodes. **Lymph node-negative** means that cancer has not spread to the lymph nodes. See Lymph Nodes.

Lymphatic System
The network of lymph nodes and vessels in the body.

Lymphedema
Swelling due to poor draining of lymph fluid that can occur after surgery to remove lymph nodes or after radiation therapy to the area. Most often occurs in the upper limbs (arm, hands or fingers), but can occur in other parts of the body.

M

Macrobiotics (Macrobiotic Diet)
Integrative or complementary dietary therapy that includes a mostly vegetarian, organic food diet with certain methods of food preparation.

Magnetic Resonance Imaging (see **MRI**)

Malignant
Cancerous.

Mammary Duct (see **Duct**)

Mammary Duct Ectasia
A benign (not cancer) breast
condition resulting from
inflammation (swelling) and
enlargement of the ducts behind
the nipple. Often there are no
symptoms, but calcifications seen
on a mammogram may point
to its presence. No treatment is
needed if the woman is not having
symptoms (burning, pain or
itching in the nipple area).

Mammary Glands
The breast glands that produce
milk.

Mammogram
An X-ray image of the breast.

Margins
The rim of normal tissue
surrounding a tumor that has been
surgically removed. A margin is
clean (also known as uninvolved,
negative or clear) if there is only
normal tissue (and no cancer cells)
at the edges. Clean margins show
the entire tumor was removed.
With involved (also known as
positive) margins, normal tissue

does not completely surround
the tumor. This means the entire
tumor was not removed and more
surgery is needed to get clean
margins.

Mastectomy
Surgical removal of the breast.
The exact procedure depends
on the diagnosis. See Total
Mastectomy and Modified Radical
Mastectomy.

Mastitis
An inflammation (swelling) of the
breast usually occurring during
breastfeeding. Symptoms include
pain, nipple discharge, fever,
redness and hardness over an area
of the breast.

Mean
The average of a group of
numbers.

Mean Survival Time
The average time from the start
of treatment (or diagnosis) that
people in a study stay alive.

Median
The middle value (50th percentile)
of a group of numbers.

Medical Oncologist
A physician specializing in

the treatment of cancer using chemotherapy, hormone therapy and targeted therapy.

Melatonin
Hormone made by the pineal gland in the brain. It is an important part of the body's internal timing system.

Menarche
The first menstrual period.

Menopausal Hormone Therapy (Postmenopausal Hormone Use, Hormone Replacement Therapy)
The use of hormone pills containing estrogen (with or without progestin) to ease symptoms of menopause.

Menopause
The ending of the normal menstrual cycle in women. It occurs most often in the late forties or early fifties.

Meta-Analysis
A method for taking the results reported in a group of studies and averaging them to come up with a single, summary result.

Metabolism
The chemical process whereby drugs and food are broken down by the body.

Metastasis
Spread of cancer to other organs through the lymphatic and/or circulatory system.

Microcalcifications
Small, clustered deposits of calcium in the breast that may be seen on a mammogram. These may or may not be related to breast cancer.

Microvascular Surgery
Surgery that involves connecting small blood vessels.

Modified Radical Mastectomy
Surgical removal of the breast, the lining of the chest muscles and some of the lymph nodes in the underarm area. Used to treat early and locally advanced breast cancer.

Molecular Breast Imaging (see **Nuclear Medicine Imaging of the Breast**)

Monoclonal Antibodies
Immune proteins that can locate and bind to cancer cells. They can be used alone or they can be used to deliver drugs, toxins or radioactive material directly to tumor cells. Trastuzumab (Herceptin) is an example of a monoclonal antibody used to treat breast cancer.

Mortality Rate
Number of deaths in a given group of people over a certain period of time.

MRI (Magnetic Resonance Imaging)
An imaging technique that uses a magnet linked to a computer to make detailed pictures of organs or soft tissues in the body.

mTOR (Mammalian Target of Rapamycin) Inhibitors
A class of targeted therapy drugs that may increase the benefit of hormone therapy. Everolimus (Afinitor) is an example of an mTOR inhibitor.

Multifocal Tumors (Multicentric Tumors)
One or more tumors that develop from the original breast tumor.

Multimodality Therapy
Use of two or more treatment methods (such as surgery, radiation therapy, chemotherapy, hormone therapy and targeted therapy) in combination or one after the other to get the best results.

Mutation (Gene Mutation)
Any change in the DNA (the information contained in a gene) of a cell. Gene mutations can be harmful, beneficial or have no effect.

N

Naturopathy (Naturopathic Medicine)
A medical system based on a belief in using natural elements to maintain health and to help the body heal itself. It includes therapies such as nutrition and massage.

Needle Localization (see **Wire Localization**)

Neoadjuvant Chemotherapy (Induction Chemotherapy, Primary Chemotherapy, Preoperative Chemotherapy)
Chemotherapy used as a first treatment. Often used for large or locally-advanced cancers to shrink tumors before surgery.

Neoadjuvant Hormone Therapy
Hormone therapy used as a first treatment. Often used for large or locally-advanced cancers to shrink tumors before surgery.

Neoadjuvant Therapy (Preoperative Therapy)
Chemotherapy or hormone therapy used as a first treatment. Often used for large or locally-advanced

cancers to shrink tumors before surgery.

Neoplasia
Abnormal growth.

Neoplasm
Excess number of cells in a mass that can be either benign (not cancerous) or malignant (cancerous).

Nested Case-Control Study
A case-control study done within a prospective cohort study. The major advantage of a nested case-control study over a regular case-control study is the exposure of interest (for example, diet or alcohol use) is measured before any of the participants have disease, making it less subject to bias.

Nipple-Sparing Mastectomy
A breast reconstruction procedure that removes the tumor and margins as well as the fat and other tissue in the breast, but leaves the nipple and areola intact.

Node-Negative (Lymph Node-Negative)
Cancer that has not spread to the lymph nodes. See Lymph Node Status.

Node-Positive (Lymph Node-Positive)
Cancer that has spread to the lymph nodes. See Lymph Node Status.

Non-Invasive
1. In treatment, describes a procedure that does not penetrate the skin (or any body opening) with a needle or other instrument.

2. In breast cancer pathology, describes a cancer that has not spread beyond the ducts or lobules where it began (see Carcinoma in Situ).

Nonpalpable
Describes a breast lump or abnormal area that cannot be felt but can be seen on an imaging test (such as a mammogram).

Normal Tissue
Cells that are cancer-free.

Nuclear Medicine Imaging of the Breast (Molecular Breast Imaging)
A technique under study for use in the early detection of breast cancer. Nuclear medicine imaging uses short-term radioactive agents given through an IV. Cancer cells absorb these agents and can be imaged with a special camera. Nuclear

medicine imaging is not a standard breast cancer screening tool. Breast-specific gamma imaging and scintimammography are types of nuclear medicine imaging.

Nucleus
The part a cell that contains the genetic material DNA. Nuclei is the plural of nucleus.

O

Observational Study
A research study where participants live their daily lives as usual and report their activities to researchers.

Odds Ratio
A measure reported in case-control studies that describes the increase (or decrease) in disease risk related to a risk factor. An odds ratio is interpreted in the same way as a relative risk, though it is calculated differently.

Oncologist
The physician in charge of planning and overseeing cancer treatment.

Oophorectomy
Surgical removal of the ovaries.

Opiate
A drug that contains opium or a substance made from opium and is used to treat pain.

Opioid
A drug that does not contain opium or any substances made from opium, but is used to treat pain.

Osteoporosis
A condition marked by a loss of bone mass and density that causes bones to become fragile.

Out-of-Network Provider
Any health care provider or medical center (hospital or other treatment center) that is not part of a particular group health plan or health maintenance organization (HMO).

Overall Survival (Overall Survival Rate, Survival)
The percentage of people alive for a certain period of time after diagnosis with a disease (such as breast cancer) or treatment for a disease.

P

Paget Disease of the Breast (Paget Disease of the Nipple)
A rare cancer in the skin of the

nipple or in the skin closely surrounding the nipple that is usually, but not always, found with an underlying breast cancer (ductal in situ carcinoma or invasive breast cancer). In these cases, the tumor grows from underneath the nipple and breaks out onto the surface of the nipple.

Palliative Therapy (Palliative Care, Palliation)
Care focused on relieving or preventing symptoms (like pain) rather than treating disease.

Palpable
Describes a breast lump or abnormal area that can be felt during a clinical breast exam.

Palpation
To examine, using the hands and fingers.

PARP (polyADP-ribosepolymerase) Inhibitors
A class of targeted therapy drugs that block an enzyme involved in DNA repair (called PARP enzyme).

Partial Mastectomy (see **Lumpectomy**)

Pathologic Response
A measure describing how much of the tumor is left in the breast and lymph nodes after neoadjuvant (before surgery) therapy. The pathologic response gives some information about prognosis. A complete pathologic response means there is no invasive cancer in the tissue removed during breast surgery.

Pathologist
The physician who uses a microscope to study the breast tissue and lymph nodes removed during biopsy or surgery and determines whether or not the cells contain cancer.

Peri-Menopause
The time in a woman's life prior to menopause when menstrual periods become irregular and some menopausal symptoms may begin.

Peripherally Inserted Central Catheter (PICC)
A small tube used to deliver medicine to the body through a vein. Instead of being reinserted for each use, a PICC is left in place to allow access for a long period of time (weeks to months).

Permanent Section
A method used in diagnosis. Thin slices of tissue are processed and put on a slide so that a pathologist can study them under a microscope. These sections are of better quality than frozen sections.

Perometer
A device that uses infrared light beams to measure limb volume.

Personalized Medicine
Using information about a person's genes, the tumor's genes, molecular characteristics of the tumor and the environment to prevent, diagnose and treat disease (such as the use of targeted therapies).This may also be known as precision medicine.

PET (Positron Emission Tomography)
A procedure where a short-term radioactive sugar is given through an IV so that a scanner can show which parts of the body are consuming more sugar. Cancer cells tend to consume more sugar than normal cells do. PET is sometimes used as part of breast cancer diagnosis or treatment, but is not used for breast cancer screening.

Pharmacogenomics (Pharmacogenetics)
The study of the way genes affect a person's response to drugs to help predict which drugs may offer him/her the most benefit.

Phenotype
A characteristic in a person that results from the interaction between his/her genes and his/her environment.

Phyllodes Tumor
A rare sarcoma (cancer of the soft tissue) in the breast.

Pituitary Gland
A part of the brain that controls growth and other glands in the body, such as the ovaries.

Placebo
An inactive medicine sometime used to have a comparison to a new drug in a clinical study. May be called a "sugar pill."

Pooled Analysis
A method for collecting the individual data from a group of studies, combining them into one large set of data and then analyzing the data as if they came from one big study.

Positron Emission Tomography (see **PET**)

Postmenopausal Hormone Use (see **Menopausal Hormone Therapy**)

Precision Medicine
Using information about a person's genes, the tumor's genes, molecular characteristics of the tumor and the environment to prevent, diagnose and treat disease (such as the use of targeted therapies). This may also be known as personalized medicine.

Predictive Factors
Factors (such as hormone receptor status) that help guide treatment for a specific cancer case.

Predispose
To make more at risk for a disease.

Premenopausal Women
Women who have regular menstrual periods.

Premium (Insurance Premium)
The cost of insurance coverage for a certain period of time.

Preoperative Chemotherapy (see **Neoadjuvant Chemotherapy**)

Prevalence Rate
The proportion (percentage) of people in a population who have a certain disease, behavior or characteristic at a defined point in time.

Prevention
Steps taken to lower the risk of a disease.

Primary Chemotherapy (see **Neoadjuvant Chemotherapy**)

Primary Tumor
The original cancer.

Progesterone
A hormone made by the body that is important in menstrual cycles and pregnancy. May be made in a laboratory (called progestin) and used in birth control pills, menopausal hormone therapy and other types of hormone treatment.

Progesterone Receptor
Specific proteins on cells that progesterone hormones attach to. A high number of progesterone receptors on a breast cancer cell often means the cancer cell needs progesterone to grow.

Progestin
Any substance (laboratory-made or natural) that has some or all of the effects of progesterone in the body.

Prognosis
The expected or probable outcome or course of a disease (the chance of recovery).

Prognostic Factors
Factors (such as tumor type, size and grade) that help determine prognosis.

Progression
The growth or spread of cancer, with or without treatment.

Progression-Free Survival
The length of time a person lives with cancer (such as metastatic breast cancer) before the cancer grows or spreads.

Proliferative
Rapidly growing and increasing in number.

Prophylactic Mastectomy
Preventive surgery where one or both breasts are removed in order to prevent breast cancer. When both breasts are removed, the procedure is called bilateral prophylactic mastectomy.

Prospective Study
An observational study that follows people forward in time. See Cohort Study.

Prosthetic (Breast Prosthetic, Prosthesis)
An artificial breast form that can be worn under clothing after a mastectomy.

Protocol
An outline or plan for the use of an experimental drug, treatment or procedure in cancer therapy or diagnosis.

Punch Biopsy
Removal of a small circle of skin (with a special instrument called a punch or trephine) to be tested for cancer cells.

Q

Quadrantectomy
Surgery where one quadrant or 25 percent of the breast is removed. See Lumpectomy.

Quality of Care
Measures of how well breast cancer is treated and how well a person is cared for during and after treatment.

Quality of Life
A measure of a person's well-being and his/her overall enjoyment of life.

Quartiles
Categories of an exposure (like body weight or exercise) based on four equal parts of the total number of people in the study.

Quantiles
Categories of an exposure (like body weight or exercise) based on equal parts of the total number of people in the study. When the total number of people is divided into thirds, the categories are called tertiles. When the total number of people is divided into quarters, the categories are called quartiles.

R

RAD (dose of radiation)
Short for "radiation absorbed dose." This term describes the amount of radiation absorbed by the tissues. One RAD is equal to one centigray. See Centigray.

Radial Scars (Complex Sclerosing Lesions)
A benign (not cancer) breast condition with a core of connective tissue fibers. Ducts and lobules grow out from this core.

Radiation Oncologist
A physician specializing in the treatment of cancer using targeted, high energy X-rays.

Radiation Therapy (Radiotherapy)
Treatment given by a radiation oncologist that uses targeted, high energy X-rays to kill cancer cells.

Radical Mastectomy (Halsted Radical)
Surgical removal of the breast, chest muscles and underarm lymph nodes. Used only when the breast tumor has spread to the chest muscles.

Radio-opaque
Does not allow radiation to pass through. A radio-opaque object will show up on an X-ray.

Radiologist
A physician who reads and interprets X-rays, mammograms and other scans related to diagnosis or follow-up. Radiologists also perform needle biopsy and wire localization procedures.

Radiotherapy (see **Radiation Therapy**)

Raloxifene
A drug first used to treat osteoporosis and now also used to lower the risk of breast cancer in postmenopausal women at high risk.

Randomized Controlled Trials
Studies where researchers change some participants' behavior or provide a certain therapy to see how it affects health. Participants are randomly assigned (as if by coin toss) to either an intervention group (such as one getting a new drug) or a control group (such as one getting standard treatment).

Reconstruction (see **Breast Reconstruction**)

Recurrence (Relapse) **Return of cancer.** Local recurrence is the return of cancer to the same breast or the same side chest wall. Distant recurrence is the return of cancer that has spread to other parts of the body, such as the lungs, liver, bones or brain. See Metastasis.

Regimen
A treatment plan.

Regional Lymph Nodes
In breast cancer, the axillary (in the underarm area) lymph nodes, infraclavicular (under the collarbone) lymph nodes, supraclavicular (above the collarbone) lymph nodes and internal mammary nodes. See Lymph Nodes.

Regression
The shrinking of a tumor.

Relative Risk
A measure used to describe the increase (or decrease) in risk related to a specific risk factor. A relative risk is the ratio of two absolute risks: the numerator is the absolute risk among those with the risk factor and the denominator is the absolute risk among those without the risk factor. A relative risk that is greater than one shows a factor increases risk. A relative risk that is less than one shows a factor decreases risk. And, a relative risk of one shows the factor neither increases nor decreases risk (this means the factor is not likely related to risk of the disease).

Relative Survival (Relative Survival Rate)
A measure used to compare the survival of people who have a certain disease with those who do not at a given time after diagnosis or treatment. The relative survival rate shows whether the disease shortens life. If relative survival is 100 percent at five years after treatment, there is no difference in survival between those who have the disease and those who do not five years after treatment.

Retrospective Study
A study where both the exposure (such as alcohol use) and the outcome (such as breast cancer) occur before the start of the study.

Risk (of disease)
Probability (chance) of disease developing in a person during a specified time period.

Risk-Benefit Ratio
The relationship between the possible (or expected) side effects and benefits of a treatment or procedure.

Risk Factor
Any factor—from a lifestyle choice (such as diet) to genetics to an environmental exposure (such as radiation)—that increases or decreases a person's risk of developing a certain disease.

RNA (Ribonucleic Acid)
A molecule made by cells containing genetic information that has been copied from DNA. RNA performs functions related to making proteins.

S

Saline
A saltwater solution similar to that found in IV fluids. Saline can be used to fill a breast implant.

Scalp Cooling
The use of a cap filled with a chilled substance during chemotherapy. Scalp cooling is under study as a technique for reducing hair loss due to chemotherapy.

Schedules
The different combinations and timing for chemotherapy and other drugs.

Sclerosing Adenosis
Small, benign (not cancer) breast lumps caused by enlarged lobules. The lumps may be felt and may be painful.

Scintimammography
(see **Nuclear Medicine Imaging of the Breast**)

Screening
A test or procedure used to find cancer or a benign (not cancer) condition in a person who does not have any known problems or symptoms.

Screening Mammogram
A test used to find early signs of breast cancer in a woman who does not have any known breast problems or symptoms.

Second Primary Tumor
A second breast cancer that develops in a different location from the first. This is different from a local recurrence, which is the return of the first breast cancer.

Selection Criteria
In a summary research table, the specific standards (such as study design and number of participants) a study has to meet to be included.

Selective Estrogen Receptor Modulator (SERM)
A drug that can either block the effects of estrogen or behave like estrogen, depending on the part of the body being treated. Tamoxifen and raloxifene are SERMs.

Sensitivity
The proportion (or percentage) of people who truly have the condition of interest who test positive for that condition.

Sentinel Node Biopsy
The surgical removal and testing of the sentinel node(s) (first axillary node(s) in the underarm area filtering lymph fluid from the tumor site) to see if the node(s) contains cancer cells.

Silicone Gel
Medical-grade, solid form of silicone used for breast implants. Silicone implants can mimic the feel of a natural breast better than saline implants.

Simple Mastectomy (see **Total Mastectomy**)

Skin-Sparing Mastectomy
A procedure that surgically removes the breast, but keeps intact as much of the skin that surrounds the breast as possible. This skin can then be used in breast reconstruction to cover a tissue flap or an implant instead of having to use skin from other parts of the body.

Sonogram (see **Ultrasound**)

Specificity
The proportion (or percentage) of people who truly do not have the condition of interest who test negative for the condition.

Stage of Cancer (Cancer Stage)
A way to indicate the extent of the cancer within the body. The most widely used staging method for breast cancer is the TNM system, which uses Tumor size, lymph Node status and the absence or presence of Metastases to classify breast cancers.

Staging (Cancer Staging)
Doing tests to learn the extent of the cancer within the body (the cancer's stage 0 to IV). Knowing a cancer's stage helps determine what treatment is needed and how effective this treatment may be in getting rid of the disease and prolonging life.

Standard Treatment (Standard of Care)
The usual treatment of a disease or condition currently in widespread use and considered to be of proven effectiveness on the basis of scientific evidence and past experience.

Statistical Significance
Describes whether or not the result of a study is likely due to chance. A statistically significant result likely shows a true link between a risk factor and breast cancer.

Stereotactic Needle Biopsy
Core needle biopsy done with the use of stereotactic (three-dimensional) mammography guidance.

Stereotactic Mammography
Three-dimensional mammography used to guide a needle biopsy.

Supraclavicular Lymph Nodes
The lymph nodes above the clavicle (collarbone). See **Lymph Nodes**.

Surgeon
Physician who performs any surgery, including surgical biopsies and other procedures related to breast cancer.

Surgical Oncologist
A physician specializing in the treatment of cancer using surgical procedures.

Survival (see **Overall Survival** and **Relative Survival**)

Survivor (Breast Cancer Survivor)
A person living with breast cancer (from the time of diagnosis).

Survivorship
The emotional and physical health, life and care of a breast cancer survivor from the time of diagnosis until the end of life.

Systemic (Adjuvant) Treatment
Treatment given in addition to surgery and radiation to treat breast cancer that may have spread to other parts of the body. It may include chemotherapy, targeted therapy and/or hormone therapy.

T

Tamoxifen (Nolvadex)
A hormone therapy drug (taken in pill form) used to treat early and advanced stage breast cancers that are hormone receptor-positive. These breast cancers need estrogen to grow. Tamoxifen stops or slows the growth of these tumors by blocking estrogen from attaching to hormone receptor in the cancer cells.

Targeted Therapy
Drug therapies designed to attack specific molecular agents or pathways involved in the development of cancer. Trastuzumab (Herceptin) is an example of a targeted therapy used to treat breast cancer.

Tertiles
Categories of an exposure (like body weight or exercise) based on three equal parts of the total number of people in the study.

Therapeutic Touch
An integrative or complementary therapy where trained practitioners enter a semi-meditative state and hold their hands just above a person's body to sense energy imbalances due to illness. Healing energy is then said to transfer to the person.

Thermography
An imaging technique that uses infrared light to measure temperature differences on the surface of the breast. The U.S. Food and Drug Administration (FDA) and the American College of Radiology do not view thermography as a valuable breast cancer screening method.

Tissue
A group or layer of cells.

Tomosynthesis (see **Breast Tomosynthesis**)

Total Mastectomy (Simple Mastectomy)
Surgical removal of the breast but no other tissue or nodes. Used for the treatment of ductal carcinoma in situ and, in some cases, breast cancer recurrence. Also used in prophylactic mastectomy.

Trastuzumab (Herceptin)
A drug that is a specially made antibody that targets cancer cells with a lot of the protein called HER2/neu on their surfaces. When attached to the HER2/neu protein, trastuzumab slows or stops the growth of the cancer

cells. Trastuzumab is used to treat HER2/neu-positive breast cancer. Herceptin is the brand name for trastuzumab.

Triple Negative Breast Cancer
A breast cancer that is estrogen receptor-negative, progesterone receptor-negative and HER2/neu-negative. These factors limit treatment choices. Most triple negative tumors are basal-like tumors. These breast cancers tend to be aggressive and are more common in African American women.

Tumor
An abnormal growth or mass of tissue that may be benign (not cancerous) or malignant (cancerous).

Tumor Grade
Describes how closely cancer cells look like normal cells. Grade 1 tumors have cells that are slow-growing and look the most like normal cells. Grade 3 tumors have cells that are fast-growing and look very abnormal. Grade 2 tumors fall in between grade 1 and grade 3.

Tumor Marker
A substance found in blood that may be a sign of metastatic breast cancer. Tumor markers are found in both normal cells and cancer cells, but they are made in larger amounts by cancer cells. A tumor marker may help indicate metastatic breast cancer treatment activity. The term tumor marker may also be used more broadly to refer to characteristics of tumor cells such as hormone receptors.

Tumor Profiling (Gene Expression Profiling)
Tests that give information about thousands of genes in cancer cells. Specific genes (or combinations of genes) may give information useful in prognosis and in making treatment decisions.

Two-Step Procedure
Biopsy and further surgical treatment done at two separate times.

Tyrosine-Kinase Inhibitors
A class of drugs that target enzymes important for cell functions (called tyrosine-kinase enzymes). These drugs can block tyrosine-kinase enzymes at many points along the cancer growth pathway.

U

Ultrasound (Sonogram)
Diagnostic test that uses sound waves to make images of tissues and organs. Tissues of different densities reflect sound waves differently.

Usual Hyperplasia
A benign (not cancer) breast condition where breast cells are growing rapidly (proliferating). The proliferating cells look normal under a microscope. Although usually hyperplasia is not breast cancer, it increases the risk of breast cancer.

V

Vaginal Atrophy (Atrophic Vaginitis)
Vaginal dryness.

W

Wire Localization (Needle Localization)
Insertion of a very thin wire into the breast to highlight the location of an abnormal area so that it can be removed during biopsy or lumpectomy.

X

X-ray
Radiation that, at low levels, can be used to make images of the inside of the body. For example, a mammogram is an X-ray image of the breast. At high levels of radiation, X-rays can be used in cancer treatment.

———————————————

*Parts of this glossary were adapted from the National Cancer Institute's *Dictionary of Cancer Terms* and the American Cancer Society's *Cancer Glossary*.

**Glossary terms relating to radiation therapy adapted from the Joint Center for Radiation Therapy's *Glossary of Terms*

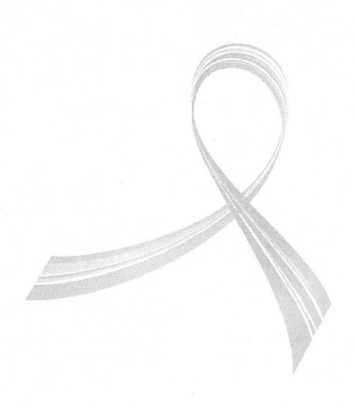

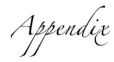

Appendix

APBI Consensus Statement,
American Society for Radiation Oncology (ASTRO)

Factors	"Suitable" group	"Cautionary" group	"Unsuitable" group
Patient factors			
Age, y	≥60	50 to 59	<50
BRCA1/2 mutation	Not present	NA	Present
Pathologic factors			
Tumor size, cm	≤2†	2.1–3.0†	>3†
T stage	T1	T0 or T2	T3 or T4
Margins	Negative by at least 2 mm	Close (<2 mm)	Positive
Grade	Any	NA	NA
LVSI	No‡	Limited/focal	Extensive
ER status	Positive	Negative§	NA
Multicentricity	Unicentric only	NA	If present
Multifocality	Clinically unifocal with total size ≤2 cm‖	Clinically unifocal with total size 2.1 to 3.0 cm‖	If microscopically multifocal >3 cm in total size or if clinically multifocal
Histology	Invasive ductal or other favorable subtypes**	Invasive lobular	NA
Pure DCIS	Not allowed	≤ 3 cm in size	If >3 cm in size
EIC	Not allowed	≤ 3 cm in size	If >3 cm in size
Associated LCIS	Allowed	NA	NA
Nodal factors			
N stage	pN0 (i⁻, i⁺)	NA	pN1, pN2, pN3
Nodal surgery	SN Bx or ALND††	NA	None performed
Treatment factors			
Neoadjuvant therapy	Not allowed	NA	If used

We hope this guide has helped you through whatever stage you are in, and that we have answered all your questions. For an extensive and wonderfully put together glossary, we recommend the website of the Susan G. Komen® organization: ww5.komen.org.